Vegan Cookbook for Athletes: Plant Based High Protein Recipes to Improve your Workout

The book with the specific diet to get healthy muscle in bodybuilding, fitness and sports

ROBERT JONSON

PLANT BASED PROTEIN

CONTENTS

PLANT BASED PROTEIN

INTRODUCTION

The most important step is to ensure sufficient protein intake, because it is vital to building new muscles. Since products such as beef, dairy and eggs largely consists of protein— while being low in alternative nutrients such as sugar, vitamin C, folate and potassium — individuals on an animal diet that wish to build muscle and energy sometimes simply consume more of their familiar foods, while supplementing with a protein shake or two.

Things are a little different for people starting from plant-based diets, in part because 'protein' wouldn't be the first ingredient to recall when they think of 'vegetarian' or 'vegan' food. They may just think of a salad which merely includes spinach, onions, cucumber and perhaps carrots — which does make for a high-protein bowl.

Naturally, in places where meat is rare, protein can be found in the form of beans, peas, lentils, tofu, peanuts, other nuts and seeds, etc. Consequently, 'developed' countries, rarely consume any of the above listed foods daily and consider plant-based foods as low-protein. Hence the problem people are constantly bombarded with on a plant-based diet – "Where are you getting your protein from?" Luckily, the plant world has an abundance of protein foods, and people who want to achieve body mass and strength on a plant-based diet just need to teach themselves about the right ingredients to include in their daily diets.

There is no scientific basis for the belief that plants have insufficient protein and that plant protein sources are "inferior". What scientific research can confirm now is the correct amount of protein (animal or plant) required to optimize and/or improve size and strength. While most people need only eat around 0.8 grams of protein per kilogram of body weight (g/kg) per day— or 0.36 grams per pound (g/lb.) — to maintain good health, focusing on muscle gain and strength has consistently demonstrated that substantially more protein is required.

Current research indicates that most sports require 1.2-2.0 g/kg of protein for performance, with endurance athletes at the bottom of the scale, while the upper end consists of bodybuilders and power athletes. If your aim is to up muscle mass and strength rapidly, as much as 2.2 g/kg of protein consumption gives promising results.

It's worth remembering that those eating a large amount of protein, despite its origins, utilize processed protein to achieve higher protein consumption levels. Unsurprisingly, eating protein at higher amounts and frequently compromises other nutrients — like carbohydrates — and doubling-down on protein can potentially undo progress, as we'll address below. Since the bodies and aspirations of all are different, personal exploration is the best way to achieve.

Doing the Numbers

Many desiring to gain muscle are not experienced bodybuilders or powerlifters, we have chosen a range between 1.6-1.8 g/kg (0.73-0.82 g/lb.)— deemed more than enough for most competitors — to provide some sample measurements.

Use your weight (in kilograms) and subtract by 1.6 - 1.8 or use your weight in pounds (subtracting 0.73-0.82 lbs.) to note the amount of you need to consume per day to live within this range. For example, if you are 77kg/170lbs., you need 123-139 grams of protein a day.

If you take five meals a day, divide your total protein requirements by five to calculate the amount per meal of protein you need each time. As per the above example, 123-139 grams of daily protein requirements can be divided by five to bring about 25-28 grams of protein per meal. You can of course consume more protein for one meal and less for another, because your actual daily intake is paramount.

Practically speaking, vegan food options would include protein rich options like peanut butter sandwiches, chili, a tofu, plant-based meatballs with spaghetti, or a protein shake with bananas and berries. Check out our section on Recipes for a wide range of protein-dense salads, smoothies, and snacks.

Nutrition Isn't Everything

Though having enough calories and nutrition is vital to gaining muscle and energy, carbohydrates do help in such objectives by giving the power needed to complete intensive workouts and provide valuable brain control. Enabling helping us stay sharp during physical endurance activities on workouts and competitions.

Evidence reveals low-carbohydrate like the trendy low-carb ketogenic diets, continue to hinder objectives in training and may delay or even obstruct increases in muscle and power. In a scientific study run over eight weeks, participants consumed identical calories and protein, found that some of those consuming normal carbohydrates managed to gain an average of 2.9 pounds of lean muscle mass whereas those eating low-carbohydrates ketogenic meals acquired 0 pounds of lean muscle mass.

Sacrificing carbs for protein will slow progress, even without going low in carb. Another study focused on rugby players with body compositions being the same amongst both groups, demonstrates that those who ate more plant-based diets with sufficient carbohydrates garnered muscle mass of less than 6 pounds whereas those who eat more protein-based diets gained only 1 pound.

Further recent studies suggest that the intake of carbohydrates within a range of 5-7g/kg — or 2.3-3.2 g/lb. — is efficient for optimizing gains. Multiply you weight (kilograms) by 5-7, or your weight (pounds) by 2.3-3.2 to measure your daily carb needs to help in height and strength improvements.

Additional Advantages

Plants contain a myriad of nutrients — including enzymes and phytochemicals — hence a plant-based diet is useful to preserve and defend new body tissues. As illustrated in 'The Plant-Based Advantage', some of these benefits include:

1. Increased energy: giving us the confidence and endurance to exercise

2. Increased blood flow: providing more oxygen to muscles but also flows

increased nutrients needed to prevent and cure injuries.

3. Reduced inflammation: speeding up exercise recovery times. Reducing unnecessary inflammation can also improve healing from injuries, taking you back to exercise so much faster.

4. Increased muscle capacity, which helps us to pull out more reps. One test investigating the impact of eating plants rich in nitrate found that participants were able to lift 19% per cent more total weight.

As epitomized by the body builders and power athletes — including world-record keeping Strongman Patrik Baboumian, American record-holding Olympic weightlifter Kendrick Farris, and the Tennessee Titans defensive line — it is not only important to establish and retain strength and power on a plant-based basis; but rapidly becoming another new reality across many sports.

CHAPTER ONE

IMPORTANCE AND STRENGTHS OF A PLANT-BASED DIET IN SPORT

Plant based diets play an important role in cardiovascular health which is important for athletes requiring stamina. Yet, even well-trained athletes are at risk for heart disease, as research done in 2017 finds. The study found that there were coronary plaques in 44 per cent of middle-aged and older distance riders or athletes. A low-fat, vegetarian diet is the most scientifically proven successful nutritional method for removing the plaque. A plant-based diet also tackles other main atherosclerosis factors including dyslipidemia, increased blood pressure, increased body weight and diabetes.

Plant-based diets are usually high in carbohydrate content, which can also give performance benefits. Carbohydrates are the primary source of energy during aerobic exercise and a high intake of carbohydrates enhances stamina. However, in a 2016 Ironman triathlete study, it was found that less than half registered as meeting the recommended intake of carbohydrates for athletes exercising for 1-3 hours within 24 hours.

Furthermore, the researchers believe that a plant-based diet enhances athletic performance and growth by increasing blood flow and tissue oxygenation and decreasing oxidative stress and inflammation. A diverse intake of citrus, vegetables, nuts, and legumes along with an added vitamin B12 fuels endurance athletes with all the necessary nutrients including protein, calcium, and iron. In these metabolic aspects, athletes can benefit by adopting a plant-based diet in terms of:

- Reducing body fat and encourages leaner body composition.

- Increasing carbohydrates in cereals, legumes, and root crops to enhance glycogen content in muscle cells and increase endurance.
- Increasing blood flow to body tissues and oxygen.
- Reducing oxidative damage in fruits and vegetables that are high in antioxidants by fighting free radicals.

HOW MUCH PROTEIN DO WE NEED?

How many grams of protein do we need in a day? For a woman it's about 0.5 to 1 gram per pound that you weigh. This range seems to be a general consensus. Luckily, the amount of protein needed is not hard to calculate. For example, a 130-pound woman needs 65 grams of protein in a day to maintain a balanced diet. Building muscle, requires the women to consume 130 grams of protein per day.

On the other hand, a man's protein intake should be 0.8 to 1.5 grams per pound that he weighs. Therefore, a 175-pound man should consume about 140 grams to maintain health and 263 grams if he is trying to really bulk up. Bodybuilders and pro-athletes often add protein supplements on top of protein-rich diets. Aside from animal-based protein powders vegans have the option of using vegetable based ones like pea protein.

Moderating your protein intake per meal is also beneficial. This is because there is a limited amount of protein the body can process each time.
This generally runs in amounts of 30 grams per meal, which your body needs several hours to digest. With our modern diet habits, this protein requirement should not be difficult to achieve.

Athletes should do further research as their protein needs surpasses that of non-athletes., Supplementing with processed protein like powders should do the trick of adding extra protein levels with eating yourself silly. Don't forgot to drink lots of water!

Seitan, Tofu, and Tempeh!

A staple to today's vegan diet, seitan, tofu, and tempeh are an abundant source of protein that fulfills hunger well. These products are vegetable based and have been eaten for centuries, but still beloved today.

Let's Talk Seitan

Seitan is 100% plant-based and is extremely versatile in terms of textures and flavors. It can be prepared into any shape required and prepared to suit any dish. The texture is modified through the mix and kneading techniques used.

Seitan is readily available in more stores, listing vital wheat gluten as the top ingredient. Observe for additives and preservatives. The good news is that seitan can be cooked at home due to the simple ingredients list and each of preparation. It is also affordable, often costing around $2.00 for 2 pounds, which is reasonable for its simplicity.

The last chapter of this book is titled "Let's Make Seitan." You'll find multiple recipes with different flavors and cooking methods.

Tofu Is Versatile

For centuries, tofu has been a delicacy and has only in recent decades become a household item. It is no flavor profile, but also as versatile as seitan.

The two most bought forms include silken and regular. Silken tofu has a creamy texture which allows it to lend richness to soft desserts and savory soup.

Tofu that is firmer is called regular tofu and is also readily available in supermarkets. It's bland flavor allows it to absorb marinades yet. It may be beneficial to take the time to press the tofu further. Soft blocks of regular tofu need to be drained, and medium, firm, and extra-firm tofu need to be drained and pressed. Inside this book are some recipes on how to prepare tofu.

A beginner's dish to try is scrambled tofu. You can add so many things to scrambled tofu, and it makes for a filling and High protein breakfast with very little effort. Tofu can also be prepared with a crisp outer and soft interior. For example, see the recipe "Fried dried tofu and peanut sauce". Marinated tofu can add flavor more easily, and marinated tofu revitalizes the dish. In extreme cases, silken tofu can be used to add high protein to recipes such as puddings and shakes.

How to Press Tofu

There are several ways to press tofu. Firstly, open the package and drain away the water. Then stack many paper towels on a dinner plate. Place the tofu on the paper towels and add more paper towels on top of the tofu. Put another plate on top of those towels. Now weigh it down with heavy cans or an iron skillet. The paper towels will soak up the liquid as it is being pressed. Alternately, you can buy a tofu press, which may make the process simpler with 2 hard layers with which to place the tofu, along with tightening screws. The whole process will take less than 30 minutes.

Tempeh, A Little Something Extra

Like tofu, tempeh is derived from soybeans as well, though it is prepared differently. The main difference is the presence of whole beans that have been fermented. The taste is acquired, however marinates can mask it. Prepare it to your liking – it's very versatile! Getting tempeh in 'original flavors' allows you to season to your taste.

BENEFITS OF A VEGAN DIET

<u>Healthy plant power without cholesterol</u>
Foods with animal ingredients are often considered unhealthy. It may be due to the mostly unhealthy preparation, but also due what animal products consist of. Substances that are problematic to health such as cholesterol, saturated fatty acids or purines, are increasingly found in animal products, while they are present in much smaller quantities or not at all in plants. In addition, many health-promoting ingredients, such as fiber and phytochemicals, are only present through plants.

<u>No risk foods in sight</u>
Those who attend food safety training will learn that food is divided into groups by the

Health Department and assessed according to risk. Eggs, meat and fish are considered to be risky foods, and when they are prepared, increased safety requirements must be met as they are more susceptible to contamination. With one exception (sprouts), vegetable foods are not on this list. Your plant-based meal prep is therefore longer-lasting and can also do without cooling for much longer.

<u>Never get tired of healthy secondary plant substances</u>
It is highly important to have a regular consumption of vegetables and fruits as the baseline for the implementation of healthy eating. Beans and pulses, vegetables and fruits provide numerous natural nutrients for the body to flourish.

The food groups also contain phytochemicals that influence various metabolic processes. Various health-promoting effects are attributed to secondary plant substances with benefits including the immune system stimulation, lower blood pressure and expansion of blood vessels. In addition, plant substances achieve neurological anti-inflammatory and antibacterial effects.

According to some studies, the regular consumption of vegetables and fruits can reduce the risk of high blood pressure, lower coronary heart disease and stroke. There are also signs that regular fruit and vegetable consumption can prevent weight gain. Perfect reasons to make your meal prep plant based!

<u>Animal protein versus vegetable protein</u>

Protein is not the same as the 'protein' we're accustomed to. The former is a macronutrient and is indispensable for a balanced diet, since the human body cannot produce proteins or amino acids itself. In the past, protein was a synonym for meat and is therefore still largely considered as stemming from animal origins.

Nowadays, 'protein' is an omnipresent hot topic and seems more important than ever. Whether marketed as 'protein muesli', 'protein bars' or 'protein curd', marketing departments come up with novel catchphrases to sell their products. The days when only bodybuilders talked about protein and amino acids are long gone and an increasing number of people are acutely aware that there is a difference between vegetable and animal proteins.

But what's the difference and what does that mean for your plant-based meal preps? Vegetable protein sources on average provide more valuable ingredients than animal alternatives. For example,

Vitamin B is readily available in hemp along with being a rich source of calcium, potassium, iron and magnesium. Generally, all types of legumes provide B vitamins, folate and other minerals such as iron, magnesium and zinc.

Cover nutrients

It is obvious to most people that eating lots of vegetables and fruits is healthy. However, many are unsure whether it is actually possible to cover all essential nutrients with plant-based meal prep. At this point, we can clearly say from our own experience: YES! All nutrients requirements, such as iron, calcium and magnesium, can be covered with plants. Only B12 needs to be supplemented! Contrary to many opinions, B12 does not naturally occur in meat.

In animals, B12 is also artificially supplemented. Therefore, the following applies to plant-based meal prep; keep an eye on vitamin B12 levels. However, this also applies to people who eat animal products. It is also worth taking a look at vitamin D3 and vitamin K2 (regardless of the diet)! This is related to the year-round light and sun conditions in western Europe.

But back to plant-based meal prep – with a bit of know-how, all nutrients can be covered with plants and if you eat a varied diet, you don't have to worry about whether you are consuming all the nutrients. Yet another reason to give plant-based meal preps a chance in the future!

Pre-programmed taste explosion

Your taste buds also benefit from a change in diet! Especially when you start to focus on plant-based food, you will be pleasantly surprised at what the culinary journey has in store for you. Suddenly, you will discover a variety of otherwise neglected vegetables and fruits, cereals, vegetable milk and nutmegs. The preparation of plant-based dishes often arouses creativity and the spirit of discovery in the kitchen and in the supermarket. Many report that their taste buds become more sensitive after eating and that they experience more intense tastes. We've also had this experience whereby through the plant-based diet, we have relived the familiar taste.

Stay healthy with plant-based foods

Many people find entry into the plant-based diet due to health problems. In the case of numerous clinical pictures and complaints, a plant-based diet is recommended by doctors. Cancer patients are often advised to leave out milk products. Heart sufferers are advised not to eat meat.

People with acne or neurodermatitis are also often advised not to consume milk products. A wholesome plant-based diet can also have a positive effect on blood, cholesterol and blood pressure values. If done correctly, the plant-based diet and plant-based meal prep can relieve symptoms and be used as a preventive measure. Some report having reached their ideal weight and positive effects on their digestion after changing their diet.

<u>Improved sleep</u>
Good sleep is essential, especially in a busy everyday life. Your body and mind need to regenerate at night and recharge your batteries. Perhaps you might experience insomnia or irregular sleep patterns occasionally. At this point, a plant-based diet comes in handy as many types of vegetables and nuts contain vitamin B6, tryptophan and magnesium which have a positive effect on sleep.

<u>Goodbye midday low</u>

Animal fats strain the body, especially at warm temperatures, because they have to use a lot of energy to digest them. The digestion of meat uses so much of our energy that we would like to sleep after devouring a hearty roast. This tiredness is known to many as the midday low. If you design your meal prep to be plant-based, you will quickly notice that your energy levels are sustained especially in midday. So if you easily tired after your lunch, definitely try to keep your meal prep plant based in the future.

Ability to regenerate

Regeneration could also be interpreted as "relaxation" of sorts. The ability to regenerate is understood to mean the potential of humans to recover after physical and psychological stress. For example, a plant-based diet can help regulate body weight. The "strength-to-body weight" can be influenced favorably, which improves sporting performance. The high proportion of valuable micronutrients in a balanced plant-based diet is another reason why performance and the ability to regenerate can be improved, highlighting another benefit of the plant-based diet.

TOP VEGAN SOURCES FOR PROTEIN

All nuts, grains, vegetables, fruit, and seeds have protein. Here is a list of some ingredients that rank highest in protein.

Vegetables and beans	Serving Size	Protein
Alfalfa Sprouts	½ cup	14

		grams
Artichoke Hearts	½ cup	4 grams
Asparagus	1 cup	3 grams
Black Beans	½ cup	8 grams
Black-Eyed Peas	½ cup	8 grams
Broccoli	1 cup	4 grams
Brussels Sprouts	1 cup	3 grams
Chickpeas	½ cup	7 grams
Corn	1 cup	4 grams
Edamame	½ cup	8 grams
Green Beans	1 cup	8 grams
Kale, uncooked	1 cup	4 grams
Kidney Beans	½ cup	8 grams
Lentils, cooked	½ cup	9 grams

Mushrooms, uncooked	1 cup	4 grams
Peas	1 cup	8 grams
Pinto Beans	½ cup	8 grams
Potatoes	1 cup	4 grams
Soymilk	1 cup	8 grams
Spinach, uncooked	1 cup	5 grams
Sun-Dried Tomatoes	½ cup	3 grams
Sweet Potato	1 cup	5 grams
Tempeh	½ cup	10 grams
Tofu	½ cup	10 grams
TVP (Textured Vegetable Protein), cooked	¼ cup	11 grams

Grains	Serving Size	Protein
Amaranth	1 cup	7 grams
Buckwheat, uncooked	1 cup	6 grams
Oats, uncooked	1 cup	6 grams
Seitan, cooked	1 cup	30 grams
Sprouted Grain Bread	2 slices	10 grams
Teff	1 cup	14 grams
Wild Rice, cooked	1 cup	7 grams
Seeds and Nuts	Serving Size	Protein
Almond Butter	2 tablespoons	7 grams

Almonds	1 cup	7 grams
Cashews	¼ cup	10 grams
Chia Seeds	2 tablespoons	5 grams
Hemp Milk	1 cup	5 grams
Hempseed	2 tablespoons	8 grams
Peanut Butter	2 tablespoons	8 grams
Peanuts	¼ cup	9 grams
Pepitas (pumpkin seeds)	¼ cup	8 grams
Pistachios	¼ cup	6 grams
Quinoa	1 cup	8 grams
Tahini	2	8 grams

	tablespoons	
Walnuts	½ cup	6 grams
Additions	Serving Size	Protein
Nutritional Yeast	2 tablespoons	8 grams
Spirulina	2 tablespoons	4 grams

So, let's get started with some satisfying, high-protein recipes that will help keep you going throughout the day while keeping you strong and healthy.

CHAPTER TWO
VEGAN BASED PROTEIN RECIPES

PROTEIN POTLUCK SPECIAL

Active Time: 10 minutes
Cook Time: 25 minutes
Total Time: 35 minutes
Yield: 8 servings

Protein: 36 grams per serving

Comfort food for the whole party! Whether for your family or made as a dish to go, this high-protein meal is the whole package.

INGREDIENTS

- 1 pound of lentils
- 1 bay leaf
- 1 tablespoon extra-virgin olive oil
- 1 cup finely chopped onion
- 1 green bell pepper, diced
- 2 carrots, finely chopped
- 3 Roma tomatoes, diced
- 1 teaspoon paprika
- 1 teaspoon ground cumin
- ½ teaspoon garlic powder
- ½ teaspoon onion powder
- 1 teaspoon coconut sugar
- ½ teaspoon salt

INSTRUCTIONS

1. Put the bay leaf and lentils in a big saucepan and cook according to package directions.

2. Heat oil whilst the lentils cook over medium-high heat in a very large skillet. Add the onions and bell pepper and sauté for 10 minutes. Add the remaining ingredients and sauté for 5 minutes. Add the lentils, stir, and cook for 5 minutes to heat through.

BLACK BEAN AND LENTIL SUPER BURRITOS SLOW COOKED

Active Time: 15 minutes
Cook Time: 8 hours
Total Time: 8 hours 15 minutes
Yield: 6 servings

Protein: 21 grams per serving (2 burritos)

These super easy burritos are spicy with lots of texture. The addition of avocados and black olives makes for a hearty meal.

INGREDIENTS

- 2 15-ounce cans diced tomatoes
- ¼ cup salsa
- 2 15-ounce black beans cans
- 1 cup brown rice
- ½ cup corn, fresh, frozen, or canned
- 2 tablespoons taco seasoning
- 1 teaspoon ground cumin
- 1 teaspoon salt
- 2 peppers (chipotle) in adobo sauce, finely chopped
- 2½ cups vegetable broth
- ½ cup lentils
- 12 whole wheat tortillas
- Additional toppings, such as more salsa, avocado or guacamole, and black olives

INSTRUCTIONS

1. Add the tomatoes, salsa, beans, rice, corn, taco seasoning, cumin, salt, chipotles, and broth to a slow cooker. Stir and cover. Boil slowly for 8 hours or if you want it faster for about 4 hours.

2. Add the lentils for the last 40 minutes of cooking. Continue cooking until the lentils are tender. The rice remains dry and soft with no water. This is the filling.

3. Lay out the tortillas and place about 1/3 to ½ cup (for a very large burrito) of the filling on each tortilla. Spread the filling down through the center of the tortilla. Fold each end about 1½ inches over the point edge of the beans. Then turn the long edge of the tortilla upwards. Once you have that strategy you would like to use on these, go straight ahead.

4. Stack up with more sauce, avocado or guacamole, and black olives to eat.

LOADED SWEET POTATO BURRITOS

Active Time: 15 minutes
Cook Time: 20 minutes
Total Time: 35 minutes
Yield: 6 servings

Protein: 19 grams per serving

The spicy and sweet contrast in these burritos really hits the spot. This is an updated classic, and you can fill up your tortillas as full as you like.

INGREDIENTS

- 1 tablespoon coconut oil
- 1 sweet potato, peeled and diced
- 8 ounces mushrooms, sliced
- ¾ cup diced red onion
- ¾ cup diced red bell pepper
- 1½ cups Steamed Seitan Smoky Nuggets
- 1½ teaspoons chili powder
- ½ teaspoon garlic powder
- ¼ teaspoon ground cumin
- 2 cups baby spinach, torn small
- 6 whole wheat or sprouted grain tortillas

INSTRUCTIONS
1. using an average heat, heat up oil with a huge skillet. Add the sweet potato, mushrooms, onion, and bell pepper. Sauté for 15 minutes. Add the seitan, chili powder, garlic

powder, and cumin, and cook for 5 more minutes. Add the spinach and cook just a minute or so until wilted.

2. If the tortillas are stiff, such as sprouted grain, then you can warm them in a microwave for 10 to 15 seconds. This will make them easier to roll.

3. Spoon about 1 cup of sweet potato mixture down the center of each tortilla. Roll up. Cut in half for easier handling.

SEITAN NUGGETS ROTELLE

Active Time: 10 minutes
Cook Time: 20 minutes
Total Time: 30 minutes
Yield: 6 servings

Protein: 20 grams per serving

Getting a family meal on the table in under 30 minutes, especially when you're serving comfort food to the max.

INGREDIENTS

- 3 cups Rotelle pasta
- 1 tablespoon extra-virgin olive oil
- ½ cup chopped onion
- 2 cups Steamed Seitan Smoky Nuggets, cut into bite-size pieces if necessary
- 2 cloves garlic, finely chopped
- 1 15-ounce can of diced tomatoes
- ½ teaspoon Italian seasoning
- ½ teaspoon salt
- ¼ teaspoon ground black pepper
- Scallions, for garnish (optional)

INSTRUCTIONS

1. Cook Rotelle according to directions on the package.
2. Meanwhile, heat the oil in a large skillet over medium-high heat. Add the onion and seitan and sauté for 10 minutes until the onion is translucent. Ensure you cook for about one minute after adding the garlic. Add the diced tomatoes, Italian seasoning, salt, and pepper. Bring to a boil then flip and simmer for 5 minutes. Add the cooked Rotelle. Heat through for 5 minutes.
3. If you'd like, garnish with the scallions.

BROCCOLI STIR-FRY WITH SEITAN AND CASHEWS

Active Time: 10 minutes
Cook Time: 20 minutes
Total Time: 30 minutes
Yield: 2 servings

Protein: 43 grams per serving

A sweet and tangy sauce combined with veggies and cashews makes this an impressive dish. Serve over sticky jasmine rice for the perfect finish.

INGREDIENTS
- 1 cup jasmine rice
- 2 cups broccoli, stems peeled and diced, florets cut into bite-size pieces
- ½ cup tamari
- 2 tablespoons rice vinegar
- 2 tablespoons maple syrup
- ½ teaspoon ground ginger
- ¼ teaspoon garlic powder

- 1 red bell pepper, diced
- 2 tablespoons cornstarch or potato starch
- ¾ cup Pressure Cooker Thai Nuggets
- ½ cup raw cashews

INSTRUCTIONS

1. Add the rice and transfer 2 cups of water to a medium pot. Bring to a boil, cover, reduce heat and cook for about 20 minutes or until water is absorbed and the rice is soft.

2. In the meantime, add water to a medium-sized pot using a steamer and boil. Add the broccoli to the fill and steam with boiling water for 5 minutes. Remove from steamer and set aside.

3. In an average container, put together and mix the tamari, ¼ cup plus 2 tablespoons water, vinegar, syrup, ginger, and garlic powder.

4. Add 1 tablespoon sauce mixture to a large skillet. Turn the heat up to medium high and add bell peppers. Sauté for 5 minutes. Add the broccoli and cook for 5 minutes. Push the vegetables to the side and add cornstarch to the liquid. Leaving on medium-high heat, stir for 1 minute. Mix all together and add seitan nuggets and cashews. Cook to heat through for about 3 minutes. 5. Serve over the jasmine rice.

WHITE BEAN STEW WITH CHIPOTLE LINKS

Active Time: 15 minutes
Soaking Time: 8 hours
Cook Time: 2 hours 20 minutes
Total Time: 10 hours 35 minutes
Yield: 6 servings
Protein: 27 grams per serving

This stew is an all-time favorite. It has fresh carrots and corn off the cob, and the plant-based chipotle links give it a sensational taste and texture.

INGREDIENTS

- 1 pound of navy beans
- 1 cup Steamed Seitan Chipotle
- 2 tablespoons extra virgin olive oil
- ½ cup diced onion
- 2 carrots, peeled and chopped
- 2 cloves garlic, finely diced
- 2 15-ounce cans fire-roasted tomatoes
- 2 cobs of corn, kernels cut from the cob
- 1 cup vegetable broth * 1 teaspoon basil
- 1 teaspoon hot sauce, such as Tabasco (omit if you don't like spicy; you can put it on the table instead)

INSTRUCTIONS

The Night Before Cooking

1) Place the beans in a big pot and cover with water. Swallow your hand in the water and pick up some floating beans or not looking good. Drain the beans. Place the beans back in the large pot. Fill about 4 inches above the beans with water. Let it soak up overnight on the counter.

The 2nd day

2) Drain the beans and cover them with 2 to 3 cm of fresh water. Cover and add to a boil. Turn the heat down to low medium and boil for around 1 and half to 2 hours, partially covered. At cooking time, turn a several times, however, ensure that the temperature remains in a decent simmer and that the beans are filled with water. When you can flatten one with your fingers the beans are finished.

3) When the beans are almost done, brown the seitan links on all sides. Remove from the pan and cut into about ¾-inch pieces.

4) With a big Skillet start heating over a low heat, add oil and add the chopped onion and carrots and sauté for 10 minutes. Add the garlic and cook for 1 more minute.

<u>To Finish</u>

5) Remove water from the beans and then transfer to the big pot. Now add and boil the tomatoes for ten minutes. It will be soupy. Add the corn, broth, basil, and hot sauce and bring to a boil. Turn down the heat and simmer another 10 minutes.

FRIED HOISIN TOFU WITH PEANUT SAUCE–TOUCHED UDON

Active Time: 20 minutes
Marinating Time: 30 minutes
Cook Time: 15 minutes
Total Time: 1 hour 5 minutes
Yield: 2 servings

Protein: 33 grams per serving
Marinated tofu is very well processed in this recipe. The outside is light and crisp, and the inside is soft. If you haven't eaten udon, now is your chance.

INGREDIENTS

- ½ cup of seafood sauce
- 4 tablespoons soy sauce
- 4 ounces extra-firm tofu, drained, pressed and cubed
- ¼ cup cornstarch or potato starch
- 2 tablespoons coconut oil
- 7 ounces packaged organic udon noodles
- ½ cup plus 2 tablespoons vegetable broth
- ¼ cup peanut butter

- 5 ounces baby spinach

INSTRUCTIONS
1. In a small bowl, mix hoisin and 2 tablespoons soy sauce. Add cubed tofu, toss and marinade for 30 minutes.
2. Place the corn starch on a large plate. Take out the tofu from the marinade, line it on cornstarch and throw it to cover all sides.
3. Heat the oil on a medium high heat in a large frying pan. Add tofu to hot oil and fry on all sides. Set aside.
4. Put water in a large pot and cover it. Bring to a boil and add udon. Cook for 5 minutes and drain. Set aside.
5. Add soup and peanut butter to the same saucepan and bring to a boil. Reduce heat and cook for 2 minutes, then add udon to pan. Put the sauce on the udon. Put the spinach in a pan and stir the sauce and noodles. Continue cooking on low heat for about 3 minutes until the spinach has wilted.
6. Remove from heat and split into two bowls. Place half of the tofu on each udon. Drizzle the remaining hoisin mixture from above.

ACADIAN BLACK BEANS AND RICE

Active Time: 5 minutes
Cook Time: 40 minutes
Total Time: 45 minutes
Yield: 6 servings

Protein: 16 grams per serving

Here's an updated version of that Southern classic, red beans and rice. This version is made with a variety of spices popular in Cajun country.

INGREDIENTS

- 1½ cups brown rice
- 3½ cups low sodium vegetable broth
- 1 tablespoon extra-virgin olive oil
- ½ yellow onion, chopped
- 1 green bell pepper, chopped
- 2 15-ounce cans of black beans that is rinsed and drained
- 1 clove garlic, finely chopped
- ¼ cup diced tomatoes
- 1 teaspoon parsley
- 1 teaspoon garlic powder
- 1 teaspoon onion powder
- 1 teaspoon thyme
- 1 teaspoon oregano
- ½ teaspoon cayenne pepper
- ¼ teaspoon ground black pepper
- 1 teaspoon salt

INSTRUCTIONS

1. Cook the brown rice by any method you choose. I use a rice cooker. Cook the rice with vegetable broth for this recipe.

2. using a big Skillet heat up oil to an average heat and then add the onion and bell pepper. Sauté until the onion becomes transparent, about 10 minutes. Minus the rice, add every other ingredient to the large skillet with the onion and bell pepper. Cook for 10 minutes. Add the rice and heat through.

BLUEBERRY TOFU PANCAKE

Active time: 10 minutes
Cooking time: 10 minutes
Total time: 20 minutes
Yield: 4 servings

Protein: 17 grams per serving (3 pancakes)

Eating sweet desserts in the morning is fine, especially when eating pancakes chock full of tofu and oats.

INGREDIENTS:

- 2 tablespoons flax seed meal
- 8 oz firm tofu, drained and pressed
- ½ cup of traditional oats
- 1¼ cup milk without dairy
- 1 cup general purpose flour
- 3 tablespoons of coconut sugar
- 1 teaspoon of vanilla essence
- 1 teaspoon baking powder
- 1 tsp cinnamon
- 1/2 teaspoon salt
- 1/2 teaspoon and 1 tablespoon extra-virgin olive oil, split
- ¼Cup maple syrup for serving
- ½ cup frozen blueberries, thaw, split

INSTRUCTIONS:

1. Mix flax seed meal with 6 tablespoons of water and save.

2. Add all ingredients except the blueberries and a tablespoon of oil to the food processor and mix well. Use the quick pulse button to blend 1/4 cup blueberries.

3. The leftover oil is melted in a frying pan and add ¼ cup of pancake dough to the center of the pan. When whisking one side, turn over and cook until golden. Continue until all batters are gone.

4. Sprinkle the maple syrup and the remaining ¼ cup of blueberries on top.

CHOCOLATE STRAWBERRY CHIA SEED PUDDING

Active time: 15 minutes
Chill time: 4 hours
Total time: 4 hours 15 minutes
Yield: 2 servings

Protein: 16 grams per serving

Get your fruit and protein with this breakfast on the run. Make this pudding recipe the night before and prepare a breakfast stuffed with simple fruits. Preparation time is only a few minutes.

INGREDIENTS:
- 1 cup milk without dairy
- 1/3 cup date
- ½ Cup strawberries (for garnish, additional)
- 2 tablespoons cocoa powder
- 1/2 teaspoon vanilla essence
- ¼Cup Ground Chia Seed
- 3 tablespoons of raw
- 2 tablespoons maple syrup
- For shaving chocolate and garnish (optional)

INSTRUCTIONS:
1. Add milk and date to the blender. Mix until smooth. Add strawberries, cocoa powder, vanilla, chia seeds, hemp seeds and maple syrup. Mix well. Pour into two cups, then cool for at least 4 hours.
2. If necessary, decorate the cut chocolate and strawberries.

BROCCOLI VEGETABLE DIPPER

Active time: 10 minutes
Cooking time: 25 minutes
Total time: 35 minutes
Yield: 6 servings

Protein: 6 grams per serving (2 patties)

Please enjoy vegetables. These dippers are small putties that can be picked up with your finger. Eat as it is or soak it in your favorite sauce. Party food!

INGREDIENTS:
- ¾Lentils
- 2 cups broccoli florets, fresh
- 1 tbsp chia seed
- Shredded carrots in cup
- ¼ teaspoon garlic powder
- ¼ teaspoon parsley
- 1/2 teaspoon salt
- ¼ teaspoon ground black pepper
- ¼ teaspoon onion powder
- ¼ teaspoon dried oregano
- ¼ 1 teaspoon of dried basil
- ¾ cup breadcrumbs, split
- 1 tbsp extra virgin olive oil

INSTRUCTIONS:
1. Rinse the lentils and drain. Put the lentils in a medium to large pot. ½Pour a cup of water. Bring the pot over high heat to a boil. When the water boils, lower it to medium and cook for 20 minutes or until the lentils are soft. All water must be absorbed. Set aside.
2. In the meantime, add water to a medium-sized pan also placed with a steamer and bring to boil. Attach the

broccoli to the replace and steam for 10 minutes in boiling water. Remove from the steamer and set aside.

3. Mix the ground chia seeds with 3 tablespoons of water in a small bowl.

4. Put all ingredients except the crumbs in the cup into the food processor. It has a friable texture and is processed until it binds well. Divide the mixture into 12 pieces. Roll each piece into a ball and flatten it on the putty. Coat each putty on both sides with the remaining crumbs.

5. Heat the oil to medium height in a medium frying pan and burn the putty on both sides for 3 minutes.

6. Serve dairy-free chipotle mayonnaise or other favorite spicy dip sauce.

RAINBOW VEGGIE PROTEIN PINWHEELS

Active time: 20 minutes
Total time: 20 minutes
Yield: 6 servings

Protein: 9g per serving (2 windmills)

Lay vegetables on a bed of hummus and crushed tempeh and wrap everything in a perfect holder, a green spinach tortilla. Even those who are not fond of vegetables will want to eat.

Material:

- ¼ Cup Hummus
- ¼ Cup tempeh, crushed with a food processor
- Two large spinach tortillas
- Red pepper sliced cup
- ¼ cup sliced yellow pepper

- 1 carrot, sliced
- Very thin sliced cup of purple cabbage

procedure:
1. Mix hummus and tempeh.
2. Put the tortilla. Spread the hummus mixture in a thin layer over the surface of each tortilla and stop 1 inch from the edge. Place a thin strip of each of the four vegetables next to the hummus mixture.
3. Roll each tortilla firmly and cut it sideways into a windmill. You can use nail pic branches if needed, but Hummus will help them stick at the edges.

MINI PEPPER WITH STUFFED TEMPEH CHICKPEAS

Active time: 20 minutes
Total time: 20 minutes
Yield: 6 servings

Protein: 9 grams per serving (2 peppers)

Colorful mini peppers wrap these protein-laden appetizers in small packages. Chickpeas and tempeh are just the beginning of a flavorful mix.

INGREDIENTS:
- 12 oz multicolor sweet mini pepper
- 2 oz canned chickpeas, drain, rinse
- ¾Cup tempeh, chopped
- ½ cup dairy free mayonnaise
- ¼Cup cider vinegar
- 1 teaspoon mustard

- 3 sliced green onions
- 1 tsp salt
- ¼ teaspoon cayenne pepper

INSTRUCTIONS:

1. Cut off the end of the pepper stem. Slice vertically. Remove any species inside. Set aside.
2. Put all remaining ingredients into the food processor. Pulse 4-5 times. Chickpeas should be thick. Remove the blade and stir so that the mixture is well mixed.
3. Pack half the chickpea mixture in half. Serve on a plate.

SLOW COOKER MAPLE BREAKFAST LINKS

Slow Cooker Size: 6 quarts
Active Time: 20 minutes
Cook Time: 6 hours
Total Time: 6 hours 20 minutes
Yield: 4 cups or 32 small links

Protein: 22½ grams per serving

These tender and sweet links can be sliced for multiple recipes. Freeze the seitan for a quick meal anytime.

INGREDIENTS

- 2 cups vegetable broth
- 1½ cups vital wheat gluten
- ½ cup chickpea flour
- 2 teaspoons ground sage, divided
- ¼ teaspoon onion powder
- ¼ teaspoon garlic powder
- 1 teaspoon salt
- ¼ cup tomato sauce
- 2 tablespoons maple syrup

- 2 tablespoons ketchup
- 1 teaspoon coconut oil

INSTRUCTIONS

1. Put the broth and 2 cups water in slow cooker. Turn to low. Add the gluten, flour, sage, onion powder, garlic powder, and salt to a large bowl. Mix well.

2. In a separate small bowl, add ½ cup water, tomato sauce, maple syrup, ketchup, and oil. Mix well.

3. Put a hole in the middle of dry mixture and pour in the tomato sauce mixture. Start to stir. This comes together quickly. Squeeze in one hand and let it go through your fingers about 10 times. Start to knead in the bowl. It is a wet mixture but will start to become elastic. Knead for about 3 minutes for a softer and tender breakfast link. The longer you knead, the more elastic it becomes. I keep it all in the bowl for kneading. It is much easier to clean up.

4. Pinch off small chunks and then roll between the palms of your hands, pretty quickly, back and forth. This will make thirty-two small links. You really can't form pretty links, but they will work fine in any recipe you make. Alternatively, you can make fifteen larger links. The larger size would change each link to 15 grams protein.

5. Place the links in the liquid in the slow cooker. Cover and cook on low for 6 hours. They will grow in size as they cook.

6. Remove from the slow cooker and let cool. Put it in the fridge for up to Five days and use when appropriate. They freeze really well, with or without their liquid.

SLOW COOKER VERSATILE SEITAN BALLS

Slow Cooker Size: 6 quarts
Active Time: 15 minutes
Cook Time: 6 hours
Total Time: 6 hours 15 minutes

Yield: 3 cups or 34 balls

Protein: 30 grams per serving (½ cup)

These little round balls add so much flavor and texture to your hardy dishes. They make a fantastic foundation for marinara sauce submarine sandwiches, too.

INGREDIENTS
- 1½ cups vital wheat gluten
- ½ cup chickpea flour
- 1 tablespoon mushroom powder
- ½ teaspoon dried oregano
- ½ teaspoon onion powder
- ¼ teaspoon garlic powder
- ¼ teaspoon nutmeg
- ¼ teaspoon ground ginger
- ¼ teaspoon ground cloves
- ¼ teaspoon ground sage
- ½ teaspoon salt
- ½ cup tomato sauce, divided
- 1 teaspoon liquid smoke
- 1½ cups vegetable broth, divided

INSTRUCTIONS
1. Mix the gluten, flour, mushroom powder, oregano, onion and garlic powders, nutmeg, ginger, cloves, sage, and salt in a large bowl.
2. In a small bowl, add ¼ cup tomato sauce, ¼ cup water, liquid smoke, and ½ cup vegetable broth. Mix well.
3. Put a hole in the middle of the dry ingredients and pour in the tomato sauce mixture. Mix well and start to knead. Knead for 1 minute or until the dough becomes mildly elastic. You will see the dough slightly pull back as you are kneading, and it will be a bit sticky. Pour remaining ¼ cup

tomato sauce, 1 cup vegetable broth, and 3 cups water into the slow cooker. Stir.

4. Tear off small chunks of the dough, squeeze into a round shape, and drop into the liquid in the slow cooker. There will be forty-four balls. You can also make seventeen larger balls and cut them after cooking and cooling. Or make two logs and cut into desired shapes. Close the lid and boil for 6 hours. They will grow in size as they cook. Check at 4 hours and see if you like the texture. They will become firmer as they sit in the refrigerator.

5. Remove from the pot and let cool. Serve and Enjoy

THIN SLICES AND CRUMBLES SLOW COOKER

Active Time: 10 minutes
Cook Time: 6 hours
Total Time: 6 hours 10 minutes
Yield: 4 servings

Protein: 31 grams per serving ($\frac{1}{2}$ cup)

One large oval log is a perfect shape for slicing. You have the option of cutting the log into nuggets or you can crumble it. This versatility makes this seitan a go-to for a multitude of recipes.

INGREDIENTS

- 1¼ cups vital wheat gluten
- ¼ cup chickpea flour
- 1 tablespoon mushroom powder
- 2 tablespoon nutritional yeast
- ½ teaspoon ground sage
- ½ teaspoon salt
- ¼ teaspoon garlic powder
- ¼ teaspoon onion powder
- ¾ cup tomato sauce

- 1 tablespoon tomato paste
- 2 cups vegetable broth
- ¼ cup tomato sauce

INSTRUCTIONS

1. Add the gluten, flour, mushroom powder, nutritional yeast, sage, salt, and garlic and onion powders to a large bowl.

2. Mix tomato sauce, tomato paste, and ¼ cup plus 1 tablespoon water in a small bowl. Put both the wet mixture and dry together

3. Mix and then knead for about 2 to 3 minutes or until mildly elastic. You will see the dough slightly pull back as you are kneading, and it will be a bit sticky. Shape the seitan into a log.

4. Pour 1 cup water, the vegetable broth, and tomato sauce into a 2½- to 3-quart slow cooker. Place the log in the slow cooker or roll loosely in cheesecloth and tie each end with cotton string. It does expand when cooking, so you shouldn't roll it tight. If you don't care that the outside is a bit lumpier after being cooked, then don't bother to roll in cheesecloth. Cover slow cooker and turn to low. Cook on low for 6 hours.

5. Remove the log from the liquid and place aside to cool. Serve and keep in the refrigerator. It can also be frozen for 4 months.

STEAMED SEITAN SMOKY NUGGETS

Active Time: 10 minutes
Cook Time: 40 minutes
Total Time: 50 minutes
Yield: 4 servings

Protein: 30 grams per serving (½ cup)

These smoky, savory bites make for a flavorful addition to an endless number of recipes. Robust in flavor, this small-batch recipe is also great when used as a sandwich filler. This is a densely textured seitan.

INGREDIENTS

- ¾ cup vital wheat gluten
- ¼ cup plus 2 tablespoons chickpea flour
- 2 teaspoons garlic powder
- 2 teaspoons onion powder
- ½ cup vegetable broth
- 2 tablespoons tomato sauce
- 1 tablespoon tamari
- 1 teaspoon liquid smoke
- ½ teaspoon coconut oil

INSTRUCTIONS

1. Add the gluten, flour, and garlic and onion powders to a large bowl.

2. Add the broth, tomato sauce, tamari, liquid smoke, and oil to a small bowl and mix well. Pour the mixture over the dry ingredients and blend together. Knead for 2 minutes until elastic. You will see it pull back into a rounder shape as you knead. This is a firm dough and will not double in size while cooking.

3. Add 5 cups water to a saucepan. Bring to a boil. Place a steamer basket inside the pan and turn down the heat to simmer.

4. Use a pastry cutter to slice off irregular pieces. You can squeeze them into a ball, as best you can, or leave chunky. You can also steam as one log and cut into chunks after steaming and cooling.

5. Steam for 40 minutes.

6. Remove the seitan to cool and store in the refrigerator for up to 5 days or in the freezer for up to 4 months.

STEAMED SEITAN CHIPOTLE LINKS

Active Time: 15 minutes
Cook Time: 40 minutes
Total Time: 55 minutes
Yield: 1 cup or 4 links

Protein: 30 grams per serving (½ cup)

These spicy hot links can be fried and served as a link, or they can be sliced or crumbled. Regardless, they push so many recipes over the top. This is a small-batch recipe, so you can double the ingredients if you're looking for a larger quantity.

INGREDIENTS
- 1/3 cup plus 2 tablespoons vital wheat gluten
- 2 tablespoons chickpea flour
- 1 teaspoon garlic powder
- 1 teaspoon onion powder
- 1 teaspoon taco seasoning
- 2 tablespoons tomato sauce
- 1 teaspoon chipotle hot sauce

INSTRUCTIONS
1. Add the gluten, flour, garlic and onion powders, and taco seasoning to a large bowl.
2. Mix ¼ cup water, the tomato sauce, and hot sauce in a small bowl and mix well. Pour the liquid mixture into the dry ingredients and mix. Knead for 2 minutes until elastic. You will see it pull back into a rounder shape as you knead. This is a firm dough and will not double in size as cooking.
3. Cut into four equal pieces and roll each one into a log shape.

4. Add 5 cups water to a saucepan. Bring to a boil. Place a steamer basket inside the pan and turn down the heat. Add seitan links to the steamer basket and cover. Steam for 40 minutes

5. Remove the seitan to cool and store in the refrigerator for up to 5 days or in the freezer for up to 4 months.

PRESSURE COOKER TENDER PATTIES

Active Time: 10 minutes
Cook Time: 5 minutes
Rest Time: 1 hour
Total Time: 1 hour 15 minutes
Yield: 2 cups

Protein: 30 grams per serving (½ cup)

These patties are ready in no time with an electric pressure cooker and are super simple to make. There seems to be an infinite number of recipe possibilities for these little disks.

INGREDIENTS

- ¾ cup vital wheat gluten
- ¼ cup chickpea flour
- 2 tablespoons nutritional yeast
- ½ teaspoon dried basil
- ½ teaspoon salt
- ½ teaspoon poultry seasoning
- ¼ teaspoon garlic powder
- ¼ teaspoon onion powder
- ¼ teaspoon paprika
- 2¼ cups vegetable broth, divided
- 1 teaspoon extra virgin olive oil
- ½ teaspoon tamari

- 2 tablespoons tomato sauce

INSTRUCTIONS

1. Put gluten, flour, digestive yeast, basil, salt, chicken seasoning, garlic and onion powder, paprika in a very huge bowl.

2. Mix a cup of vegetable soup, oil and tamari in a small bowl. Combine wet amalgam and dry ingredients

3. Knead for 2-3 minutes after mixing, or until elastic. It is elastic and should be pulled back, but still flexible. Divide the dough into eight. Use your finger to quantify about 3-4 inches in diameter and narrow to putty.

4. Put in electric pressure cooker. Stir 5.1½ cups of water, 1.5 cups of vegetable soup and tomato sauce in a small bowl and pour into a pressure cooker seitan cutlet. Close the lid and make sure the top knob is sealing. Press the manual on the front of the pot. Press the button to 4 (meaning 4 minutes) and in a few seconds, the pressure cooker will click and begin to build pressure. It takes about 15 minutes to cook under pressure.

5. Leave the cutlets in the pan. They cook more because the pressure is naturally abandoned. Do not vent.

6. After about an hour, go ahead and vent. It may already be completely cooled but open the lid after all vents has been opened to check pressure. 7. Pull out the cutlets from the liquid and set aside for cooling. You can activate them immediately, integrate them into recipes, or put them in the refrigerator overnight. They are great the next day and keep them in the freezer.

PRESSURE COOKER THAI NUGGETS

Active Time: 10 minutes
Cook Time: 5 minutes
Rest Time: 1 hour
Total Time: 1 hour 15 minutes

Yield: 4 servings

Small unformed nuggets with delectable flavors come from your pressure cooker with this recipe. They have an Asian flair and can be added to just about any recipe.

Protein: 30 grams per serving (½ cup)

INGREDIENTS:
- ¾ cup plus 3 tablespoons vital wheat gluten
- ¼ cup chickpea flour
- ½ teaspoon ground ginger
- ½ teaspoon salt
- ¼ teaspoon garlic powder
- ¼ teaspoon paprika
- ¾ cup vegetable broth
- 2 teaspoons tamari, divided
- 4 teaspoons red curry paste, divided
- 1½ cups vegetable broth, divided

INSTRUCTIONS
1. Add the gluten, flour, ginger, salt, garlic powder, and paprika to a large bowl.
2. Mix ¾ cup vegetable broth, 1 teaspoon tamari, and 2 teaspoons red curry paste in a small bowl. Throw all the mixture that is wet into the mixtures that are dry.
3. Mix and then knead for about 2 to 3 minutes or until elastic. It's a very wet dough but you will see it is still elastic. It should be mildly stretchy and pull back but still pliable. Pinch off pieces of dough into very small balls, about 1 to 1½ inches in diameter. They will fatten up when cooking. Place in an electric pressure cooker.
4. Add 1½ cups vegetable broth, 1½ cups water, and 2 teaspoons red curry paste to a bowl and stir well. Pour over the nuggets in the pressure cooker. Close the lid and make sure you spin the top knob to lock. Click Manual at

pot end. Press button to 4 (that means 4 minutes). The pressure cooker will give a click and the pressure will begin to build. Building pressure, and cooking, will take about 15 minutes. Leaving the nuggets to fall in the pot. They are going to cook more as the pressure of course releases. Don't wind.

5. Go ahead and vent after about an hour. It may have already completely cooled, but vent to ensure that the pressure has been released and then open the lid.

6. Take the nuggets off the liquid and set aside to cool and eat shortly in a recipe or keep in the fridge overnight. They are great the next day or freeze them.

APPLE BROCCOLI CRUNCH BOWL

Active Time: 20 minutes
Total Time: 20 minutes
Yield: 6 servings

Protein: 9 grams per serving

Here's a bowl that's filled with everyone's favorite vegetables and fruits. Mix all the ingredients inside a bowl then pour on the slightly sweet and tangy dressing. Toss and eat!

INGREDIENTS
Bowl

- 2 medium heads broccoli (about 4 cups when chopped)
- 3choice apples that is diced
- ¼ cup diced red onion
- ½ cup raisins
- ½ cup sunflower seed kernels
- ¼ cup raw shelled hempseed Dressing

- ¼ cup cider vinegar
- ½ cup extra virgin olive oil
- 2 cloves garlic, minced
- 1 tablespoon maple syrup (you can use up to 2 tablespoons)
- ½ teaspoon salt
- ¼ teaspoon ground black pepper

INSTRUCTIONS

Bowl

1. Cut the florets from the broccoli stalks and set the stalks aside. Cut the florets into very small pieces. Place in a large bowl.

2. remove after slicing the hard external part of the skin away from the broccoli stalks to get down to the tender inside. Discard the outer skin. Cut the inside stems into matchsticks. (Or you can use a mandolin or food processor that has an attachment that will cut the stems into long strips—not grated. The aim is to have very tiny points of raw broccoli stems that retain their form Remove the florets then remove to the large mixing bowl. Stir in the apples, onions, raisins, sunflower seeds, and hempseed.

Dressing

3. Mix and stir all dressing ingredients in a medium bowl. Introduce the salad dressing, and toss. Chill to fully prepare for serving.

SMOKY TEMPEH BUDDHA BOWL

Active Time: 15 minutes
Cook Time: 35 minutes
Total Time: 50 minutes
Yield: 2 servings

Protein: 15 grams per serving

A warm and colorful lunch is something worth your time. The ingredients in this bowl act as complements to each other, with the added bonus of protein.

INGREDIENTS
Bowl

- 1 small sweet potato, chopped into bite-size pieces
- 1 tablespoon extra-virgin olive oil
- ½ teaspoon salt
- ¼ cup dry quinoa
- ½ cup vegetable broth
- 4 ounces faux bacon-flavored tempeh

Almond Curry Sauce

- 3 tablespoons almond butter
- 3 tablespoons dairy-free milk
- 1½ tablespoons tamari
- 1 tablespoon rice vinegar
- 1 tablespoon red curry paste

To Assemble

- 2½ cups baby spinach
- ½ cup chopped red bell pepper
- ½ cup chopped purple cabbage

INSTRUCTIONS
Bowl
1. Preheat the oven to 375°F.
2. Put the potatoes on the baking sheet. Put oil on the edge
3. Meanwhile, quinoa is cooking. Place the quinoa and rinse well with a sieve. Mix the quinoa and soup in a small pot. Bring to a boil, cover, and boil until simmered. Cook for 10-15 minutes or until the soup is absorbed. Remove from heat and set in cover for 5 minutes.

4. Cut the tempeh into 1/4 slices and then into cubes. Almond curry

5. In a small bowl, mix all ingredients until smooth and well mixed.

6. Fill each salad bowl with the spinach. Make a decorative rim with the spinach tips if so desired. Divide the quinoa and vegetables between the two bowls and lay in a circle: peppers, quinoa, cabbage, sweet potatoes, and lastly, tempeh. Drizzle the dressing in a circle all over.

CHOPPED CHICKPEA SALAD VEGGIE BOWL

Active Time: 20 minutes
Cook Time: 15 minutes
Total Time: 35 minutes
Yield: 2 servings

Protein: 17 grams per serving

This is a delicious dish that incorporates chickpea salad. There's lots of roughage, too, that just begs for the simple balsamic dressing.

INGREDIENTS
Quinoa

- ½ cup dry quinoa
- 1 cup vegetable broth
- Pinch of salt
- Chickpea Salad
- 1 15-ounce can chickpeas, drained and rinsed
- ¼ cup vegan mayonnaise
- 1 tablespoon nutritional yeast
- 1 tablespoon cider vinegar
- ½ teaspoon ground mustard
- 2 scallions, finely sliced

- 1 teaspoon salt
- Pinch of cayenne pepper

Dressing

- ½ cup extra virgin olive oil
- ¼ cup balsamic vinegar

To Assemble

- 3 cups chopped romaine lettuce
- ½ cup diced purple cabbage
- ½ cup diced orange bell pepper

INSTRUCTIONS

Quinoa

1. Sift the quinoa and rinse well. Mix the quinoa, soup and salt in a small pot. Bring to a boil, cover and boil down. Cook for 15 minutes or until the soup is absorbed. Turn off heat and schedule for Five minutes with cover attached. Remove the lid and put it in a fluffy small bowl to cool. Chickpea salad

2. Put all the ingredients of the chickpea salad into the food processor. Pulse 4-5 times. Chickpeas should be thick. Remove the blade and stir so that the mixture is well mixed.

Dressing

3. Mix the oil and vinegar together in a small bowl and set aside. Assembly

4. Divide the lettuce between two bowls. Lay the vegetables in decorative rows: cabbage, quinoa, bell pepper, and chickpea salad, leaving an edge of romaine lettuce. Serve with the dressing.

ROASTED ROOT VEGETABLE SALAD BOWL

Active Time: 15 minutes
Cook Time: 35 minutes
Total Time: 50 minutes

Yield: 2 servings

Protein: 24 grams per serving

Here's the perfect bowl to get a good helping of vegetables. Simply roast a few root vegetables and then chop a few more veggies to create this healthy power bowl. It's perfect with a nutty sweet tahini sauce.

INGREDIENTS
Roasted Vegetables
- 1 peeled sweet potato
- 1 parsnip, peeled and sliced into ¼-inch rounds
- 2 carrots, peeled and sliced into ½-inch rounds
- 2 tablespoons extra virgin olive oil
- ½ teaspoon salt
- Tahini Dressing
- ¼ cup tahini
- 1 tablespoon maple syrup
- 1 tablespoon lemon juice
- 1 clove garlic
- ¼ teaspoon salt
- Pinch of ground black pepper
- 3 tablespoons water

To Assemble
- ¼ cup diced red onion
- ½ cup chopped red cabbage
- 9 ounces baby spinach
- ¼ cup raw shelled hempseed
- 1 tablespoon chia seeds, black or white

INSTRUCTIONS
Roasted Vegetables
1. Preheat the oven to 375°F.

2. Place the sweet potatoes, parsnips, and carrots on a baking sheet, keeping them separated. Drizzle the oil over the top and lightly toss, still keeping the vegetables separated. Sprinkle with salt. Bake till they can be pierced with a fork or for 35 minutes. Set aside. Tahini Dressing
3. Add all the dressing ingredients to a blender and blend until smooth. Assembly
4. Prepare the salad bowls by placing half the spinach in the bottom of each bowl. Arrange all the remaining vegetables and hempseed in a circle around the edge of the bowl. Pour half of the dressing in the center of the vegetable round. Sprinkle with the chia seeds.

A TOUCH OF THE TROPICS RICE BOWL

Active Time: 15 minutes
Cook Time: 10 minutes
Total Time: 25 minutes
Yield: 2 servings

Protein: 21 grams per serving

The repertoire requires rice. A great way to enjoy many kinds of fruits and vegetables, this rice introduces the taste of the tropics.

INGREDIENTS
Bowl

- 1 peeled sweet potato that is cut into pieces
- 1 tbsp extra virgin olive oil
- 2 cups jasmine rice
- 1 pineapple, peel, core and chop to bite size
- ¼ Cup cashew nut
- 4 tablespoons raw

Sweet and Sour Sauce

- 1 tablespoon cornstarch
- ½ cup chopped pineapple
- ¼ cup rice vinegar
- 1/3 cup light brown sugar
- 3 tablespoons ketchup
- 2 teaspoons soy sauce

INSTRUCTIONS
Sweet Potato
1. Preheat the oven to 425°F.
2. Throw the oil over the sweet potato. Place them on a baking sheet and fry for 30 minutes.
3. Remove from the pan and let cool. Nice sauce and sour
4. In a small bowl, mix cornstarch and a spoonful of water, Make a deposit.
5. Pour pineapple and 1/4 cup of water into the mixer. Blend as smoothly as possible until mixing is complete.
6. Put pineapple paste, rice vinegar, brown sugar, ketchup and soy sauce in a medium-sized pan. Bring to a boil over medium heat. Attach the cornstarch mixture and cook for about 1 minute until thick. Remove from heat and set aside

Assembly
7. Put rice in each bowl below. Removes clusters of bananas, cashews, sweet potatoes, and hemp seeds, On a sweet and sour sauce

SOUTHWEST VEGGIE-PACKED SALAD BOWL

Active Time: 20 minutes
Cook Time: 25 minutes

Total Time: 45 minutes
Yield: 2 servings
Protein: 24 grams per serving

Vibrant colors fill this bowl with all the best vegetables associated with the Southwest. Add a small sweet potato and a spicy dressing and you're all set.

INGREDIENTS
Vegetables

- 1 small sweet potato, peeled and chopped in bite-size pieces
- 2 tablespoon extra-virgin olive oil, divided
- ½ cup green lentils
- ½ cup diced red onion
- ½ cup diced bell pepper, orange and yellow
- ½ cup canned kidney beans, drained and rinsed
- 1 ear corn on the cob, kernels cut off of cob
- 1 teaspoon salt

Dressing

- ¼ cup extra virgin olive oil
- ¼ cup lime juice
- 2 tablespoons maple syrup
- ¼ to ½ teaspoon hot sauce
- ½ teaspoon salt To Assemble
- 2 cups mixed lettuce ½ cup grape tomatoes, sliced in half

INSTRUCTIONS
<u>Vegetables</u>
1. Preheat the oven to 400°F.
2. Put the sweet potato on a baking sheet and sprinkle with 1 tablespoon oil and toss. Roast for about 25 minutes or until you can pierce the sweet potato easily with a fork

3. While the sweet potato is roasting, rinse the lentils. Add 1 cup water and the lentils to a medium saucepan. Cover, bring to a boil, crack lid, and turn down the heat to medium. Cook about 20 minutes or until the lentils are tender

4. Heat 1lb of oil in a saucepan on average heat. Put the onion and bell pepper together for 10minutes and sauté or until the onion is translucent. Add the kidney beans and corn and heat through. Stir in the lentils, sweet potato, salt, and set aside.

<u>Dressing</u>

5. Mix all the ingredients for the dressing and set aside.

<u>Assembly</u>

6. Divide the lettuce between two salad bowls, pulling the lettuce up higher on half of the bowl. Divide the lentil mixture between each bowl, filling up half the bowl. Lay a row of sliced grape tomatoes between the lettuce and vegetable mixture. Serve with the dressing.

SPICED CAULIFLOWER TEMPEH SALAD BOWL

Active Time: 20 minutes
Cook Time: 15 minutes
Total Time: 35 minutes
Yield: 2 servings

Protein: 20 grams per serving

Baked cauliflower comes into its own with some spices added. Marinate tempeh in a slightly tangy dressing, add a little more color and taste contrast, and you'll be in power mode in no time.

INGREDIENTS

Bowl

- 1 small head of cauliflower, cut into florets
- 2 tablespoons extra virgin olive oil
- 1 teaspoon salt
- ½ teaspoon ground cumin
- ¼ teaspoon ground black pepper

DRESSING

- ½ cup vegan mayonnaise
- ¼ cup unsweetened dairy-free milk
- 1 teaspoon lemon juice
- ¼ teaspoon garlic powder
- ¼ teaspoon onion powder
- ¼ teaspoon dill weed
- Pinch of salt
- Pinch of ground black pepper
- 8 ounces tempeh, sliced into ¼-inch-thick slices and then into small bite-size pieces
- 8 ounces baby spinach
- 1 small red onion, cut into bite-size pieces
- 2 carrots, cut into small matchstick pieces
- 1 yellow bell pepper, cut into bite-size pieces

INSTRUCTIONS

Cauliflower

1. Preheat the oven to 400°F.

2. Put the blooming cauliflower in a large mixing bowl. Sprinkle oil, salt, cumin, and ¼ teaspoon pepper. Bake about 25 minutes or until tender. Remove from the oven and set aside.

Dressing

3. While baking, mix the mayonnaise, milk, lemon juice, garlic and onion powders, dill weed, salt, and pinch of pepper in a small bowl. Place the tempeh in the dressing to marinate while the cauliflower is baking.

<u>Assembly</u>
4. Divide the spinach between two salad bowls. Make a line in the shape of an arc with each vegetable starting with the onion and continuing on with the carrots, cauliflower, and bell pepper. Remove tempeh from the marinade and add it as the final touch to the bowl. Serve with the dressing.

EDAMAME AND BROCCOLI RICE BOWL

Active Time: 20 minutes
Cook Time: 30 minutes
Total Time: 50 minutes
Yield: 2 servings

Protein: 20 grams per serving

Tahini sauce pulls this rice-based bowl all together. Each vegetable can stand on its own, but when they mingle with each other, the result is memorable.

INGREDIENTS
Bowl
- ½ cup broccoli florets
- ½ cup edamame, frozen
- ¼ teaspoon salt
- ¼ cup peas, frozen or fresh
- ½ cup chopped yellow bell pepper Tahini Sauce
- ¼ cup tahini
- 1 tablespoon lemon juice
- 1 tablespoon maple syrup
- 1 tablespoon tamari To Assemble
- 2 cups jasmine rice, cooked
- ¼ cup sunflower seed kernels
- ¼ cup raisins

INSTRUCTIONS
Bowl
1. Add water to a medium-sized pan Replace with a steamer and bring to boil. Stir in broccoli and heat in boiling water for 10 minutes. Remove from the steamer and set aside.
2. Bring 2 cups water to a boil in a small saucepan and add the edamame and salt. Boil for 5 minutes, adding the peas during the last minute. Drain and set aside.
3. Meanwhile, add 2 tablespoons water to a small skillet and heat over medium-high heat. Sauté for 10 minutes after you have added the pepper bell. Remove from the heat and set aside.
<u>Tahini Sauce</u>
4. Add all the ingredients plus 5 tablespoons water to a small bowl and blend until smooth.
Assembly
5. Add the rice to the bottom of each bowl. Divide the remaining items in half and add onto the rice in a pinwheel fashion, making sure that the greens don't touch each other for a more pleasing design.
6. Serve with the tahini sauce.

CARIBBEAN CHILI

Active Time: 30 minutes
Cook Time: 1 hour
Total Time: 1 hour 30 minutes
Yield: 4 servings

Protein: 13 grams per serving

Treat yourself to some spicy chili with a bucketful of veggies. This recipe can be served all year round because of its warmth in the winter and its summer festive vibe.

INGREDIENTS:

- 2 tablespoons coconut oil
- 1 onion, diced
- 1 green pepper, diced
- 3 Roma tomatoes, chopped
- 2 carrots, diced
- 5 ounces tomato paste
- 2 tablespoons chili powder
- 1 teaspoon salt
- 1 teaspoon ground cumin
- ½ teaspoon cinnamon
- ½ teaspoon allspice
- ½ teaspoon dried oregano
- ½ teaspoon cayenne pepper
- ¼ teaspoon garlic powder
- ¼ teaspoon garlic, minced
- ¼ teaspoon ground black pepper
- 1 oz 15 oz kidney beans, drain, rinse
- 1 corn, grain cut from cob

INSTRUCTIONS

1. In a broad skillet boil up the oil over moderate heat and add the onions and peppers. Fry for about 10-15 minutes until the onions are translucent.

2. Add tomatoes, carrots, tomato paste and 1/2 cup of water. Add spices and herbs. Bring to a boil, cover and boil for 30 minutes.

3. Add the kidney beans and corn. Cook on a low simmer for another 15 minutes.

MIXED BEANS CHILI

Active Time: 10 minutes
Soaking Time: 8 hours
Cook Time: 1 hour 30 minutes
Total Time: 9 hours 40 minutes
Yield: 6 servings

Protein: 20 grams per serving

How about some vegan chili that is comforting and full-flavored at the same time? It's made from scratch to warm your family's and your hearts.

INGREDIENTS

- 1 pound of beans, mixed varieties (you can buy premixed or mix your own)
- 1 tablespoon extra-virgin olive oil
- ½ cup diced onion
- 4 cloves garlic, finely chopped
- 4 cups vegetable broth, more if needed
- 1 28-ounce can of crushed fire-roasted tomatoes
- 1 8-ounce can tomato sauce
- 1 6-ounce can tomato paste
- 2 tablespoons vegan Worcestershire sauce
- 2 tablespoons chili powder
- 2 teaspoons ground cumin
- 1½ teaspoons dried oregano
- ¼ teaspoon ground cloves
- ½ teaspoon cayenne pepper
- 1 teaspoon salt

INSTRUCTIONS

Night before
1. Rinse beans and place in large stock pot with about 3 inches of water to soak overnight. Next morning
2. Discharge the beans and return to the stock pot.
3. Heat the oil on a medium high heat in a large frying pan. Sauté onions until translucent (approximately 10-15 minutes). Add garlic and fry for another minute. Add this mixture to the stockpot. with vegetable soup, crushed tomatoes, tomato sauce, tomato paste and Worcester sauce. Beans should be covered with a few inches of liquid. Add broth or water as needed. Stir well. Add the remaining ingredients and mix again. Cover and bring to a boil.
4. Remove the lid, reduce the heat and cook over very low heat so the liquid hardly moves. Do not replace the lid. Remove the lid for more flavor. Add some soup or water as needed (If so, re-cover, bring the heat to a boil, lower immediately and remove the cover). Make sure the heat is not too high. Cook for 1 hour until the beans are soft. If not, cook it longer. There is no need to cook for over an hour and a half.

ULTIMATE VEGGIE WRAP WITH KALE PESTO

Active Time: 30 minutes
Soaking Time: 2 hours
Cook Time: 10 minutes
Total Time: 2 hours 40 minutes
Yield: 2 servings

Protein: 24 grams per serving

Pretty in green on the inside and out. Tender broccoli and fresh veggie layers add to the flavorful kale pesto before you roll these up for your first bite.

INGREDIENTS
Kale Pesto

- ¼ cup of raw cashew nuts, soaked for at least 2 hours
- 1 cup kale, coarsely chopped with stem removed
- 1 clove garlic
- ½ teaspoon salt
- 2 tablespoons nutritional yeast
- 3 tablespoons extra virgin olive oil Wrap
- ½ cup broccoli florets
- 2 spinach tortillas
- ¼ cup grated carrots
- ¼ cup diced red onion
- ½ yellow bell pepper, diced
- 6 ounces spinach
- 2 tablespoons raw shelled hempseed
- 2 tablespoons sunflower seed kernels

INSTRUCTIONS
Kale Pesto
1. Place the cashews, kale, garlic, and salt in a small food processor. Process for about 30 seconds, add the nutritional yeast and oil and process a few more seconds until well blended. Set aside. Assembly
2. Add water to a medium-sized pan with a steamer and just get it to a boil. put in the steam the broccoli in boiling water for 10 minutes. Remove from the steamer and set aside.
3. Lay out the spinach tortillas. Divide the kale pesto between the two tortillas and spread evenly, leaving about 1 inch around all edges. Divide the remaining ingredients in half and lay out each half next to each other and down the length of each tortilla.
4. Start to roll up snugly, without tearing the tortilla. Cut each tortilla in half and serve.

SPROUT SANDWICH WITH TOFU RICOTTA

Active Time: 30 minutes
Total Time: 30 minutes
Yield: 2 servings

Protein: 26 grams per serving

A nice thick layer of homemade tofu ricotta and sun-dried tomato pesto make a terrific sandwich. Add even more veggies for a unique and delicious lunch.

INGREDIENTS
- Sun-Dried Tomato Pesto
- ¼ cup baby spinach, packed
- Fill two tablespoons of sun-dried tomatoes in oil and drain. (Save oil)
- 1 tablespoon pine nuts
- 1 clove garlic
- 2 teaspoons nutritional yeast
- Pinch of garlic powder
- ¼ teaspoon salt
- 1 tablespoon oil or reserved oil from the sun-dried tomatoes
- Tofu Ricotta
- 7 ounces extra-firm tofu, drained, pressed and crumbled
- 1 tablespoon extra-virgin olive oil
- 1 teaspoon cider vinegar
- 1 teaspoon lemon juice
- ½ teaspoon garlic powder
- ½ teaspoon onion powder

To Assemble
- 4 slices sprouted grain bread

- 1 cup alfalfa sprouts
- 1 Roma tomato, sliced
- 2 slices red onion
- Pinch of garlic powder

INSTRUCTIONS

Sun-Dried Tomato Pesto
1. In a food processor add all the ingredients starting with the spinach. Process until well blended. Tofu Ricotta
2. Place all the ricotta ingredients in a small food processor. Process until well blended. Assembly
3. Spread a thick layer of the tofu ricotta on two bread slices. Apply pesto on the other two slices of bread. Divide the sprouts, tomato, and onion and place on the ricotta. Top with the pesto slice. Slice each sandwich into fourths in triangle shapes.

PESTO AND CRISPY TOFU FLATBREAD SANDWICH

Active Time: 15 minutes
Soaking Time: 1 hour
Cook Time: 40 minutes
Total Time: 1 hour 55 minutes
Yield: 2 servings

Protein: 33 grams per serving

Multiple textures and flavors galore make this sandwich a prime recipe for regular rotation in your meals.

INGREDIENTS
Tofu

- 2 ounces extra-firm tofu, drained, pressed, and cut into 1-inch cubes
- ¼ cup vegetable broth
- 1 tablespoon tamari
- 1 teaspoon onion powder
- ¼ teaspoon salt
- ¼ cup cornstarch

Pesto
- ¼ cup raw cashews, soaked for 1 hour
- 1 cup basil, packed
- 1 clove garlic
- ½ teaspoon salt
- 2 tablespoons nutritional yeast
- 3 tablespoons extra virgin olive oil
- To Assemble
- 1 tablespoon coconut oil
- ¼ cup diced onion
- 6 mushrooms, sliced
- ¼ cup hummus
- 2 slices flatbread
- ½ cup sunflower sprouts

INSTRUCTIONS

Tofu
1. Mix together the vegetable broth, tamari, onion powder, and salt in a small bowl. Add the tofu and let marinate at least 1 hour.
2. Preheat the oven to 350°F.
3. Place the cornstarch in a medium bowl.
4. Coat marinated tofu in cornstarch. Pour it onto the baking sheet and set it. Bake 40 minutes. Flip every 10 minutes with the spatula until it golden. Pesto
5. Place the cashews, basil, garlic, and salt in a small food processor. Process for about 30 seconds. Add the

nutritional yeast and olive oil and process a few more seconds until well blended. Assembly

6. Heat the coconut oil in a skillet over medium-high heat. Add the onions and mushrooms and sauté for about 10 to 15 minutes or until onion is translucent. Remove from the heat.

7. Spread half of the hummus and pesto on each flatbread. Sprinkle remaining ingredients down the center of each flatbread. Fold each flatbread and secure it with a decorative pick.

SEITAN AND SUN-DRIED TOMATO PESTO VEGGIE SANDWICH

Active Time: 20 minutes
Cook Time: 20 minutes
Total Time: 40 minutes
Yield: 2 servings

Protein: 28 grams per serving

Thick slices of special seitan and tender cauliflower make the best sandwich when combined with pesto and spinach. After all is encased in a folded flatbread, it simply begs for a bite.

INGREDIENTS
Cauliflower

- 1 tablespoon extra-virgin olive oil
- ½ cup cauliflower florets
- Pinch of salt
- Sun-Dried Tomato Pesto

- ¼ cup baby spinach, packed
- Fill two tablespoons of sun-dried tomatoes with oil and drain. (Save the oil)
- 1 tablespoon pine nuts
- 1 clove garlic
- 2 teaspoons nutritional yeast
- Pinch of garlic powder
- ¼ teaspoon salt
- 1 tablespoon oil or reserved oil from the sun-dried tomatoes

To Assemble
- 2 slices flatbread
- 1 ounce of baby spinach
- ¾ cup Slow Cooker Maple Breakfast Links, sliced
- 2 slices red onion

INSTRUCTIONS
Cauliflower
1. Preheat the oven to 425°F.
2. Sprinkle the oil on a baking sheet. Lay the cauliflower on the oil and sprinkle with salt. Toss with your hands to get the oil dispersed onto the cauliflower. Bake for 20 minutes till it is visible the cauliflower can be pierced easily with a fork, Remove and set side. Sun-Dried Tomato Pesto
3. Mix all of the pesto ingredients and position in an average food processor, starting with the spinach. Process until well blended. Assembly
4. Lay out the flatbreads. Spread half the pesto on each flatbread. Divide the spinach, seitan, cauliflower, and onion between the flatbread slices. Fold each flatbread and secure it with a decorative pick.

PORTOBELLO MUSHROOM GYRO

Active Time: 15 minutes
Cook Time: 15 minutes
Total Time: 30 minutes
Yield: 2 servings

Protein: 16 grams per serving

Big, fat, marinated Portobello is a dream ingredient. Just wrap in flavored drops with spinach and add the best white sauce.

INGREDIENTS
Vegetables

- 2 large portobello mushroom caps
- 2 tablespoons vegan Worcestershire sauce
- 1 teaspoon ground cumin
- 1 teaspoon maple syrup
- ½ teaspoon dried oregano
- 1 tablespoon coconut oil
- ¼ cup diced red onion
- ½ red bell pepper, diced large
- Fresh White Sauce
- ½ cup vegan mayonnaise
- ¼ cup raw shelled hempseeds
- 1 tablespoon lemon juice
- ¼ teaspoon dried mint
- ¼ teaspoon dill weed

To Assemble

- 2 pita flatbreads
- 1 ounce of baby spinach

INSTRUCTIONS
Vegetables
1. Remove the stem from the mushroom and remove the gills with a spoon. throw away. Cut the mushrooms thick.

2. Mix Worcestershire sauce, cumin, maple syrup and oregano in a medium bowl. Place the mushroom slices in the marinade and marinade for 10 minutes.
3. Heat the oil on a medium high heat in a large frying pan. Add the onions and peppers and fry for 10 minutes. Add the marinated mushroom slices and fry for an additional 5 minutes. Remove from heat and cool. Fresh white sauce
4. Mix all the fresh white sauce ingredients in a small bowl and set aside. Assembly
5. Place a layer of spinach leaves on each flatbread. Spoon a fresh white sauce in the middle. Place the mixture of mushrooms and peppers on top. Fold each flatbread and secure it with a decorative pick.

VEGGIE STUFFED CALZONE

Active Time: 30 minutes
Rising Time: 90 minutes
Cook Time: 25 minutes
Total Time: 2 hours 25 minutes
Yield: 2 servings

Protein: 21 grams per serving

This homemade calzone dough is stuffed with prepared veggies and a little bit of veggie goodness. Slide it in the oven to bake for a great lunch that you deserve.

INGREDIENTS
Dough
- 1 packet dry active yeast
- 1 tablespoon extra-virgin olive oil
- ¾ teaspoon salt
- ¾ cup whole wheat pastry flour
- 1 cup unbleached all-purpose flour

Filling

- 2 cups broccoli florets
- 1 tablespoon extra-virgin olive oil
- 1 red bell pepper, diced
- 1 cup cremini mushrooms
- ½ cup diced red onion
- 4 ounces artichoke hearts in water, drained
- 2 tablespoons chopped walnuts
- ½ teaspoon dried rosemary
- ¼ teaspoon salt
- ¼ teaspoon ground black pepper
- ½ cup vegan mayonnaise or spread of your choice
- 2 tablespoons dairy-free milk
- 2 tablespoons cornmeal

INSTRUCTIONS

Dough

1. Apply oil to the inside of a large bowl and set aside. This is because the dough rises.

2. Put a cup of warm water (100-110 ° F) into another large, heated bowl (you can warm the bowl with a microwave). Stir the yeast and leave for 10 minutes. Put water, oil and salt in a cup and mix. Stir until flour is added and mixed. Not smooth.

3. Transfer to a floured counter and knead for about 4 minutes until smooth. To avoid sticking, add a little more flour. A little sticky is OK. Knead into a round-like ball. Position the dough ball in a big oiled mixing bowl and coat the dough until all surfaces are greased. Failure to do this will result in a dry crust on the outside of the ball. Cover the bowl and let it sit (from the draft) for 40-60 minutes until the dough doubles in size.

4. Divide the dough in half. Half the dough is formed into two balls and placed on a floured counter. Cover with a towel again and raise for another 20-30 minutes.

5. On a lightly powdered surface, flatten and extrude the dough with your fingers, or use a rolling pin to form two

circles of the same size (about 10 inches each). One is up and the other is down. Cover again with towels and rest for 10-15 minutes.

Filling

6. Add water to the medium-sized pan with Insert the steamer and bring to a boil. Stir in broccoli and steam in boiling water for 10 minutes. Remove from the steamer and set aside.

7. Heat the oil over medium high heat in a large frying pan. Add red peppers, mushrooms and onions and fry for 10 minutes. Add artichoke heart, walnuts, rosemary, salt and pepper and fry for another 5 minutes. Stir the broccoli and set aside.

Assembly

8. Preheat the oven to 425°F.

9. Uncover the calzone dough. Spread the mayonnaise on one dough round. Next spread the broccoli mixture, leaving about ½ to 1 inch of the edge not covered. Carefully lift the plain dough round and place on the broccoli-covered round. Press and fold the edges over. Cut a few slits in the top of the dough. Brush lightly with milk.

10. Spread the cornmeal on a baking sheet. Carefully lift the calzone onto the baking sheet. Bake for 15 to 18 minutes.

11. Cut the calzone as you would a pizza and serve.

SEITAN SLOPPY JOES

Active Time: 10 minutes
Cook Time: 20 minutes
Total Time: 30 minutes
Yield: 6 servings

Protein: 26 grams per serving

A rich barbecue sauce and enriched seitan make for a much-loved sandwich. Hold it over a plate and have a big bite. Now that's good!

INGREDIENTS

- 2 cups seitan, crumbled (Slow Cooker Log for Thin Slices and Crumbles)
- 8 ounces tomato sauce
- 1/3 cup organic ketchup
- 1 tablespoon vegan Worcestershire sauce
- 2 tablespoons red wine vinegar
- 2 tablespoons coconut sugar
- 6 toasted whole wheat buns

Instructions:

Add all of the ingredients except the buns to a large skillet. In an average heat, boil and Cook for 15 minutes. Serve on the toasted buns.

SPICED GREEN LENTIL SANDWICH

Active Time: 20 minutes
Cook Time: 10 minutes
Total Time: 30 minutes
Yield: 8 servings

Protein: 14 grams per serving

Lots of texture and wonderful flavors enhance this spiced-up sandwich. It's one of the best veggie combinations you could ask for.

INGREDIENTS

- 1 cup green lentils
- 1 small potato, to equal about ½ cup mashed potato
- ½ cup chopped onion

- 1 carrot, finely chopped in a processor
- ¾ cup old-fashioned oats
- ½ cup pepitas or sunflower seed kernels
- 1 tablespoon hempseed, toasted in shell
- 1 cup breadcrumbs
- 4 tablespoons tamari
- 1 teaspoon ground ginger
- 1½ teaspoons smoked paprika
- ½ teaspoon salt
- ¼ teaspoon ground black pepper
- 1 tablespoon coconut oil
- 8 sandwich buns

INSTRUCTIONS

1. Place 2 cups water and the lentils in a large saucepan. Cover and bring to a boil. Turn down to low and cook for 20 minutes. Drain off remaining liquid from the lentils, if any. Set the lentils aside.

2. Pierce the potato several times with a sharp knife. Wrap in a damp paper towel. Set in the microwave and cook on high for 4 minutes or until you can pinch the potato easily. Peel the potato and mash well. Set aside.

3. Heat 2 tablespoons water in a skillet over medium-high heat. Add the onion and sauté for 10 minutes. Remove from the heat.

4. Add the lentils, potato, onion, and the remainder of the ingredients to a large bowl (excluding the oil and the buns). Mix well. Form eight patties to the size of your sandwich buns.

5. Using a frying pan, heat it and fry the lentil patties on each side without crowding. 6. Spread the buns with all your favorite condiments and any other toppings of your choice. 7. You may also freeze extra patties for future meals.

BLACK BEAN PATTIES WITH CARROTS AND CORN

Active Time: 15 minutes
Cook Time: 20 minutes
Total Time: 35 minutes
Yield: 6 servings

Protein: 22 grams per serving

Treat yourself to one of the most popular sandwiches out there. An added bonus is that this version has little bits of carrots and corn.

INGREDIENTS

- 1½ cups breadcrumbs, fresh
- 2 tablespoons of chia seed or ground chia seed
- 2 tablespoons coconut oil, divided
- 1 cup diced yellow onion
- ½ cup finely diced carrot
- 1 ear of kernel and corn removed from the cob, or 1 8-ounce can corn, drained
- ½ teaspoon dried oregano
- 2 teaspoons chili powder
- ¼ teaspoon ground cumin
- 1 teaspoon salt
- 2 cloves garlic, finely diced
- 1 28-ounce can black beans, drained and rinsed
- ¼ cup sunflower seed kernels
- 2 tablespoons raw shelled hempseed
- 6 whole wheat buns
- Condiments and toppings of your choice

INSTRUCTIONS

1. Make your breadcrumbs using any leftover bread that you have. I used whole wheat but you could use sourdough and whatever else you prefer. Place bread in a food processor and process until the bread is a finely ground texture. Set aside. If you have any leftover breadcrumbs, they can be frozen for 6 months.
2. Mix the chia seeds with 6 tablespoons water and set aside.
3. Heat 1lb of oil in a big saucepan, add the onion and carrot, and sauté about 10 minutes. Add the corn and cook another 3 minutes. Add the spices and garlic to the onion and cook another minute.
4. Pat the black beans dry. When mashing and adding the remaining ingredients, you need to make sure they are not wet. In a big mixing bowl, add black beans and a mash behind a potato masher or fork. Pulse them in a food processor instead, but not too fine. Stir in the chia seed mixture. Mix in the onion mixture, breadcrumbs, sunflower seed kernels, and hempseed.
5. Make into six patties. After freeze the patties before frying
6. Fry the patties in 1 tablespoon medium-hot oil until browned on each side.
7. Serve on the whole wheat buns with your favorite toppings.

DOUBLE-DECKER RED QUINOA SANDWICH

Active Time: 20 minutes
Cook Time: 35 minutes
Total Time: 55 minutes
Yield: 3 servings

Protein: 24 grams per serving

A little preparation, and a food processor, takes you a long way in making this satisfying sandwich. Red quinoa has the same nutty taste and nutrition of its pearly cousin and it's just darn pretty.

INGREDIENTS

- ½ cup red quinoa
- 1 cup vegetable broth
- 4 large portabella mushroom caps
- 2 tablespoons coconut oil, divided
- ¼ cup finely chopped onion
- ½ cup raw pecans
- 2 green spring onions, chopped
- 2 teaspoons rice wine vinegar
- 1 teaspoon garlic powder
- 2 tablespoons nutritional yeast
- 2 tablespoons raw shelled hempseed
- ¼ cup flour
- 3 whole wheat burger buns

Toppings and condiments: lettuce, tomatoes, red onion, mustard, dairy-free spicy mayo

INSTRUCTIONS

1. Soak the quinoa, then rinse properly. Mix the quinoa in a small pot and the soup. Bring to a boil and cover, then steam. Cook for 10-15 minutes, or until it consumes the broth, remove from heat and put on cover for 5 minutes.

2. Drop gills and discard mushrooms. Chop a stem on the mushroom.

3. In a large frying pan, melt a spoonful of oil. Remove the mushrooms and onion, and fry for 10 minutes. Add the pecans and sauté for 5 more minutes. Remove from the heat and let cool.

4. Add the mushroom mixture, green onion, and vinegar to a food processor. Process until very fine. It will not be smooth.

5. move to a big bowl and mix quinoa, garlic powder, nutritional yeast, hempseed, and flour. Mix until well blended. Form into six patties the size of the burger buns.

6. Heat remaining oil in a large skillet and fry one patty at a time so that you can flip it easily. Fry until golden brown on each side.

7. Assemble the double-deckers: Lay down the bottom of the bun, add mustard, lettuce, patty, red onion, lettuce, dairy-free spicy mayo, patty, dairy-free spicy mayo, tomatoes, and top of bun.

LOADED CHICKPEA SALAD SANDWICH

Active Time: 15 minutes
Total Time: 15 minutes
Yield: 8 servings

Protein: 21 grams per serving

Here's a complete meal for your whole family. It's a big batch, it's quick to prepare, and it keeps well in the fridge or freezer.

INGREDIENTS

- 2 15-ounce cans chickpeas, drained and rinsed
- 2 15 oz cans of pinto beans, drain, rinse
- 2 tablespoons raw shelled hempseed
- 1 tablespoon vegan mayonnaise (add another tablespoon if you like it better that way)
- 1 tablespoon Dijon mustard (add another tablespoon if desired)
- 2 tablespoons lemon juice (optional)
- ¼ teaspoon garlic powder
- ¼ teaspoon paprika

- ½ teaspoon salt
- ¼ teaspoon ground black pepper
- 16 slices whole wheat bread or sprouted grain bread
- 2 avocados, sliced
- 2 ounces baby spinach

INSTRUCTIONS

1. In a large bowl, add the beans and mash. Leave a bit chunky, not completely mashed. Add the remaining ingredients except the bread, avocado, and spinach. Mix well.

2. Spread on the bread slices. Add the avocado slices and spinach. You can also keep any extra chickpea salad in your fridge for up to 5 days.

MIXED BAG CHOCOLATE WALNUT PROTEIN BARS

Active Time: 20 minutes
Cook Time: 35 minutes
Total Time: 55 minutes
Yield: 8 servings

Protein: 9 grams per serving

The long slim bars will have you happily chewing your way to daily healthy protein enrichment.

INGREDIENTS

- 3 tablespoons peanut butter
- 3 tablespoons maple syrup
- 1½ tablespoons coconut oil
- 1 tablespoon ground chia seeds
- 1¼ cups quick-cooking oats

- ½ cup walnuts
- ½ cup dairy-free chocolate chips
- 1/3 cup coconut sugar
- ¼ cup raw shelled hempseed
- 3 tablespoons protein powder
- ½ teaspoon ground cinnamon
- ¼ teaspoon salt

INSTRUCTIONS

1. Preheat the oven to 350°F.

2. Prepare an 8-inch square baking dish with parchment paper coming up on the sides on two opposite ends. Not over the top, just the sides. This makes for easier removal.

3. Add the peanut butter, maple syrup, and coconut oil to a small saucepan. Heat to melt the peanut butter and stir well. Take off heat and let cool a bit.

4. Mix the ground chia seeds and 3 tablespoons water in a small bowl and set aside.

5. Add the oats, walnuts, chocolate chips, sugar, hempseed, protein powder, cinnamon, and salt to a large bowl. Mix well. Add the chia mixture and peanut butter mixture to the bowl of dry ingredients and mix well.

6. put the mixture together in the bowl and press down with your fingers to make the mix firm and pressed into all corners.

7. Bake for 30 to 35 minutes. The bars will get harder as they cool, so don't overbake.

8. Let cool on a wire rack. To remove, grab hold of the extra parchment paper on the opposite ends of the dish and lift. Cut into bars that are about 2 inches wide and 4 inches long.

PEANUT BUTTER SNACK SQUARES

Active Time: 10 minutes

Cook Time: 20 minutes
Total Time: 30 minutes
Yield: 8 servings

Protein: 14 grams per serving (2 squares)

A double peanut whammy is served up in this recipe. All is sweetened with whipped coconut sugar and dates.

INGREDIENTS

- ½ cup coconut sugar
- 1 cup creamy peanut butter
- 1 teaspoon vanilla extract
- ¾ cup whole wheat flour
- ¼ cup garbanzo flour
- 1 teaspoon baking soda
- ½ teaspoon baking powder
- 1 cup old-fashioned oats
- ½ cup dairy-free milk
- ½ cup peanuts
- ½ cup dates, pitted and chopped small

INSTRUCTIONS

1. Preheat the oven to 350°F. Lightly grease an 8-inch square baking dish.
2. Mix the sugar and peanut butter over medium speed with a hand or stand mixer for 5 minutes. Mix the coffee in with it. Add the flours, baking soda, baking powder and mix at medium velocity. Pour in the oats and mix for a couple of seconds. This is going to be rigid. Add the milk and blend until just mixed on a medium.
3. Wrap in the peanuts and dates to make sure that everything is well set in.
4. You can use your hands to gently press the dough into the shaped platter. Bake for 15 to 20 minutes, or until golden brown is light.

5. Place to cool onto a wire rack. Cut into seventeen squares, and store in the fridge.

RICH CHOCOLATE ENERGY COOKIES

Active Time: 15 minutes
Cook Time: 15 minutes
Total Time: 30 minutes
Yield: 12 servings

Protein: 6½ grams per serving (2 cookies)

These rich energy cookies are big and chewy and a wonderful variety of ingredients goes into them. They won't remain in your cookie jar for long.

INGREDIENTS

- ½ cup dairy-free butter, softened
- 1 cup coconut sugar
- 1 tablespoon chia seeds or ground chia seeds
- 2 cups (12 ounces) dairy-free chocolate chips, divided
- 1 tablespoon instant coffee
- 1¼ cups whole wheat flour
- ½ teaspoon baking soda
- 1 teaspoon baking powder
- ½ teaspoon salt
- 2 tablespoons raw shelled hempseed
- 1 cup walnuts, chopped

INSTRUCTIONS

1. Preheat the oven to 350°F. Cut parchment paper on a baking sheet to match. put aside.
2. To pan, add butter and sugar a stand mixer. Cream on medium speed for 5 minutes or until light and fluffy.

3. Mix the chia seeds with 3 tablespoons water and set aside.

4. Melt ½ cup of the chocolate chips in a microwave or in a double boiler. Set aside to cool a bit.

5. Boil 2 tablespoons water and add instant coffee. Set aside to cool.

6. Add flour, baking soda, baking powder, and salt to a bowl. Mix well by hand.

7. Add the prepared chia seed mixture and melted chocolate to the bowl of the stand mixer. Mix well on medium speed. Add the flour mixture and keep mixing until just combined. Put away the bowl and wrap in the remaining chocolate chips, hempseed, and walnuts. Mix well.

8. Drop on the prepared cookie sheet by large, heaping tablespoons, 2 inches apart, and flatten slightly. Bake for 12 minutes.

9. Cool on a wire rack.

PROTEIN PEANUT BUTTER BALLS

Active Time: 20 minutes
Total Time: 20 minutes
Yield: 24 balls

Protein: 10 grams per serving (2 balls)

Here's an easy and healthy treat that you can pop in your mouth any time of the day. Energy-packed with only six ingredients!

INGREDIENTS
* ½ cup creamy peanut butter
* ½ cup maple syrup
* ½ cup powdered soymilk, non-GMO
* ¼ cup flaxseed meal
* ½ cup coconut flour

* ¼ cup peanuts, chopped fine

INSTRUCTIONS

1. Position the maple syrup and peanut butter in a small mixing bowl. Start to Mix. Add the powdered soymilk, flaxseed meal, and coconut flour. Mix well and roll into 24 balls. Lightly roll each ball in the chopped peanuts.
2. keep and position in the refrigerator for two weeks.

CARROT CAKE TWO-BITE BALLS

Active Time: 20 minutes
Total Time: 20 minutes
Yield: 16 balls

Protein: 8 grams per serving (2 balls)

Carrot cake! I kid you not. Everything for a carrot cake is in here, all rolled up into perfect little balls. You can roll some in coconut and leave others plain. They are so pretty.

INGREDIENTS
* 1 cup old-fashioned oats
* ½ cup almond meal
* ½ cup pecans
* 1/3 cup plus 2 tablespoons of unsweetened shredded coconut, split
* 3 medium carrots, grated
* 15 dates, pitted
* 2 tablespoons unsweetened cocoa powder
* 2 tablespoons almond butter

- 1 teaspoon ground cinnamon
- ½ teaspoon ground nutmeg
- ½ teaspoon ground ginger

INSTRUCTIONS:
1. Add the oats, almond meal, pecans, 1/3 cup coconut, carrots, dates, and cocoa powder to a food processor. Mix on high until well processed. You may need to sharpen the edge several times to confirm the dates aren't clumping. Add the almond butter, cinnamon, nutmeg, and ginger. Mix again until well mixed. Scrape down again if needed.
2. Transfer to a flat surface and make sure all is blended well. Use your hands if necessary. Remove in pieces the dough and wrap into sixteen balls. Roll the balls in additional shredded coconut, if desired.

PUMP UP THE POWER ENERGY BALLS
Active Time: 20 minutes
Total Time: 20 minutes
Yield: 32 balls

Protein: 10 grams per serving (3 balls)

No-bake treats are so easy to make. Currants are readily available they seem to have been made to be combined with pepitas, hempseed and peanut butter.

INGREDIENTS
- 1 cup old-fashioned oats
- ¾ cup almond meal
- 1/3 cup wheat germ
- ¼ cup flaxseed meal
- ¼ cup pepitas
- 2 tablespoons raw shelled hempseed
- 1 teaspoon ground cinnamon

- ¼ teaspoon ground nutmeg
- ½ cup dried currants
- ½ cup peanut butter
- 1/3 cup maple syrup
- 1 teaspoon vanilla extract
- ¼ teaspoon salt

INSTRUCTIONS

1. Mix the oats, almond meal, wheat germ, flaxseed meal, pepitas, hempseed, cinnamon, nutmeg, and currants together in a medium bowl.

2. Add the peanut butter, maple syrup, vanilla, and salt to the bowl of a stand mixer. Mix on medium speed until well combined. Pour the dry ingredients into the wet mixture. Mix on low until well combined.

3. Roll into thirty-two balls.

CHAPTER THREE

BREAKFAST RECIPES EMPTY BAKED STICKY RICE USING SEITAN

Active time: 30 minutes
Cook time: 30 minutes
Total time: 1 hour
Yield: 4 servings

Protein: 20 grams per serving

This dinner recipe is bound to knock your socks off. The sweet and spicy sauces can be made quickly and easily. There is also an option to fry it in the pan!

INGREDIENTS:
- 2 cups jasmine rice
- ½ cup soy sauce or gluten-free puddle
- 4 tablespoons maple syrup
- 4 pieces of garlic, finely chopped

- 2 teaspoons of 5 Chinese spices
- 1/2 teaspoon ginger
- 4 tablespoons white wine or rice vinegar
- 1 pound of cremini mushroom, cleanly wiped, or cut into large mushrooms in half
- 1 cup pressure cooker Thai nuggets
- ½ cup frozen peas

INSTRUCTIONS:

1. Add rice to a large pot of 2 cups of water. Cover and bring to a boil. Cook on medium heat and cook for about 20 minutes or until water is absorbed.

2. If the fryer does not have a built-in insert, insert it now.

3. Mix soy sauce, maple syrup, garlic, 5 Chinese spices, raw ginger and white wine in a small bowl and set aside.

4. Put the mushrooms in the air fryer. If you can set the temperature, set it to 350 ° F. Otherwise, just turn it on. Air fryer temperature is built-in and is always cooked at 338 ° F. Cook for 10 minutes. Open the air fryer and add seitan nuggets. If the fryer does not have a built-in self-stirrer, stir. Pour the liquid mixture and beans from above. Stir for 5 minutes.

5. Add the rice and stir well. Heat for 2 minutes. Take out Note: If you do not have a fryer, you can make this dish in a frying pan. Pre-cook jasmine rice and set aside. Combine the following six ingredients and save. Heat a tablespoon of oil in a large skillet. Add mushrooms and cook over medium high heat for 10 minutes. Pour the liquid mixture into the mushrooms. Add the peas and seitan nuggets and cook for another 5 minutes. Add the cooked rice, stir well and cook.

STACK OF ENCHILADA CASSEROLES

Active time: 30 minutes

Cook time: 1 hour
Total time: 1 hour 30 minutes
Yield: 4 servings

Protein: 14 grams per serving

There is nothing like casserole baking and this smells very good. With two different sauces, along with vegetables and tortillas, this dinner is a quadruple victory.

INGREDIENTS:
Filling

- 1 cup of diced yellow pepper
- 1 sweet peeled potato that is cut into pieces
- 1 cup diced white onion
- 1 tbsp extra virgin olive oil
- 1 tsp salt, split
- ¼ teaspoon ground black hu pepper
- 1 15 oz black beans, drain, rinse
- 2 oz tempeh, fine pulse
- 1 teaspoon cumin
- 1 tsp chili powder
- 2 garlic cloves
- 2 cups of red enchilada sauce purchased at the store
- 6 small corn tortillas White sauce
- 2 tablespoons butter without dairy
- 3 tablespoons flour
- 1½ cup milk without dairy
- Nutritional yeast 1 tablespoon

INSTRUCTIONS:
Filling

1. Preheat oven to 400 ° F.
2. Put the peppers, sweet potatoes and onions on the baking sheet. Sprinkle with oil to make sure all vegetables are coated. Position on a baking sheet after then, season with 1/2 teaspoon of salt and pepper and put in oven and roast for 15 minutes. Remove from the oven, stir and return to the oven for another 15 minutes. Check if the sweet potato can be easily pierced with a fork. If not, stir and cook for another 10 minutes. Remove from oven and set aside. Reduce oven temperature to 350 ° F.
3. Add the roasted vegetables, beans, tempeh, cumin, chili powder and garlic to a medium bowl.
4. Spread the ¼ cup enchilada sauce on the bottom of the 8-inch square glass casserole dish.
5. Cut the four tortillas into four. Place four compartments in each corner of the casserole and turn V toward the corner. Place the whole tortilla in the center. Top with a third of the vegetable mixture and spread evenly over the tortillas. Drizzle an additional 1/4 cup of enchilada sauce. Place another tortilla layer as before. Lay another layer using one third of the vegetable mixture, then add ¼ cup of enchilada sauce. Put another layer of tortilla, then put the rest of the vegetable mixture. Set the rest of the enchilada sauce aside.

White sauce
6. Melt the butter in a medium pot. Stir flour and cook for 1 minute. Add milk and heat over medium to low heat. Add nutritional yeast and continue cooking and stirring until the sauce is thickened and boiled down in about ¼ cups. Remove from heat.

Assembly
7. Pour the remaining enchilada sauce over the casserole and spread evenly. Drizzle the white sauce back and forth on the top, but do not spread. Cover with casserole dish lid or aluminum foil sheet. Bake for 30 minutes.

8. Remove the enchilada casserole from the oven and remove the foil. Sit for 10 minutes, then serve in a square.

KALE WHITE BEAN SOUP

Staying time: 8 hours
Active time: 20 minutes
Cooking time: 2 hours
Total time: 10 hours 20 minutes
Yield: 6 servings

Protein: 14 grams per serving

This is a simple and tasty recipe and provides a complete meal. Perfect for any night of the week. Let the beans all night and you're on the way.

INGREDIENTS :

- 1 pound of navy beans
- 1 tablespoon coconut oil
- Coarse onion cup
- 1 garlic, chopped
- ¼ Cup nutrition yeast
- 1 red pepper diced
- 4 chopped Roman tomatoes
- 2 cups of carrot slices
- 5 cups vegetable soup
- 1 teaspoon Italian seasoning
- 2 teaspoon salt
- 1/2 teaspoon black pepper
- 1lb of kale, coarsely chopped with stem removed

INSTRUCTIONS:

1. Put the beans in a large stock pot and cover with about 3 inches of water. Soak the beans overnight. If you want a simple way to prepare the beans instead of soaking overnight, Cover the beans in stock pot with 2 inches of water. Cover with lid and bring to a boil. Remove from heat and leave uncovered for 1 hour. Drain the beans in a colander and set aside.

2. Put the oil in the same stock pot and heat over medium heat. Add the onions and fry for about 10-15 minutes until soft and translucent. Put garlic and boil for a minute with stirring. Add 4 cups of water, beans, nutritional yeast, peppers, tomatoes, carrots, soups, Italian seasonings, salt and pepper. Cover and bring to a boil. Start the heat and boil down. Cook for about 1 to 1.5 hours until the beans are soft.

3. Add the kale and two cups of water and simmer for about 12-15 minutes until the kale is soft.

SLOW COOKER SEITAN BOURGUIGNON

Yield: 4 servings

This dinner is rich in flavors such as mushrooms, carrots and citrus. It is easy to make, and you will be amazed by its deep taste.

INGREDIENTS:

- 2 tablespoons extra virgin olive oil
- 1 cup diced yellow onion
- 1½ cup sliced carrots
- 2 tablespoons dairy-free butter, split
- 2 garlic cloves
- 2 tablespoons flour
- 2½ cup vegetable soup
- 1 tablespoon liquid smoke
- 2 tablespoons of tomato paste
- 1 cup of good Burgundy wine

- 1 bay leaf
- 1/2 teaspoon time
- 1 tsp salt
- 1 pound mushrooms, sliced
- 2 cups slow cooker versatile seitan ball, cube

INSTRUCTIONS:

1. Apply heat the oil in a big frying pan. Add the onions and carrots and fry for 10-15 minutes or until the onions are translucent. Add 1 tablespoon butter. Put garlic and boil for one minute.

2. Add small flour and stir to coat everything and cook for another minute. Make sure the flour is fully functional and the mixture is not showing any dry flour.

3. Add all ingredients from the frying pan to the slow cooker. ½ Stir with a cup of water, soup, liquid smoke, tomato paste, wine, bay leaf, thyme, and salt. Cook over low heat for 6-8 hours.

4. Approximately one hour before serving, fry the mushrooms in a large frying pan with one tablespoon of butter for about 10 minutes. Add mushrooms and citrus to the slow cooker and cook for another hour.

5. Serve alone or with noodles, potatoes or rice.

SEITAN MAPLE LINKS BREAKFAST SANDWICH

Active time: 15 minutes
Cooking time: 20 minutes
Total time: 35 minutes
Yield: 2 servings

Protein: 34 grams per serving

The soft Seitan rink from the slow cooker is the star of this hearty and savory breakfast.

INGREDIENTS:

- 1 tbsp extra virgin olive oil
- 8 oz mushrooms, sliced
- 1 tablespoon dairy-free butter
- 1 cup slow cooker maple breakfast link
- 2 English muffins, sliced
- Seasonings of choice
- ½ Avocado, slice

INSTRUCTIONS:

1. Heat up the oil over moderate heat in a large skillet. Add mushrooms and fry for about 15 minutes. Remove the mushrooms from the pot and set aside.

2. Add butter to bread over medium high heat. Add the link to the bread for a total of about 5 minutes and brown all sides. If you increase the size of the link, slice the center vertically and fry that way. The rinks are already cooked and enjoyable cold, but the sandwich is now fine.

3. While the links are brown, toast the English muffins and spread with your favorite seasoning such as Chipotle Mayo, which does not contain dairy products. Stack the fried mushrooms, rink and avocado. English muffin slice top.

VANILLA BREAKFAST SMOOTHIE

Active time: 10 minutes
Total time: 10 minutes
Yield: 1 serving

Protein: 20 grams per serving

This smoothie is perfect for a plant-based break-breakfast breakfast. Only seven materials are required and can be made in less than 10 minutes.

INGREDIENTS:

- 1 frozen banana, slice

- 1 cup vanilla almond milk
- ¼ cup old-fashioned oats
- ¼ cup raisins
- 1 tablespoon flax seed
- ¼Cinnamon teaspoon 3 tablespoons of vanilla protein powder

INSTRUCTIONS:

Add all ingredients to the blender and blend until very smooth.

TO THE POWER OF OATS FOR FOUR NIGHTS

Active time: 10 minutes
Staying time: 8 hours
Total time: 8 hours 10 minutes
Yield: 2 servings

Protein: 23 grams per serving

If you've never eaten oats overnight, here's a great recipe to entice you. It is simple and uses the ingredients that everyone likes.

INGREDIENTS:

- 3.5 cups of unsweetened almond milk
- 2 cups of traditional oats
- ¼ cup maple syrup
- 2 tablespoons of chia seeds
- 2 tablespoons unsweetened shredder coconut
- ¼ cup sunflower seed kernel
- 4 tablespoons peanut butter, split
- Sunflower seed kernel for garnish (optional)

INSTRUCTIONS:

1. Add 2 tablespoons peanut butter and all ingredients except sunflower seeds to a large bowl. Mix well. It looks very wet, but chia seeds and oats absorb some of the milk. Cover and place in the refrigerator overnight.
2. Sprinkle the existing two cups of peanut butter inside the two bowls to serve, each with oats overnight. Decorate with sunflower seeds if necessary.

WARM MAPLE PROTEIN OATMEAL

Active time: 5 minutes
Cook time: 30 minutes
Total time: 35 minutes
Yield: 2 servings

Protein: 23 grams per serving

Do you keep forgetting oatmeal? Make this recipe and you will never forget it. This oatmeal dish that is healthy, warm and slightly sweet will hum during breakfast.

INGREDIENTS:
- 1 cup steel cut oats
- 3 tablespoons of raw tbsp, split
- 3 tablespoons maple syrup
- 2 tsp cinnamon
- 1 tbsp sliver almond
- 1 tablespoon currant

INSTRUCTIONS:
1. Boil 4 cups of water in a large pot. Add steel cut oatmeal, 2 tablespoons hemp seed, maple syrup and cinnamon and bring to a boil. Reduce heat, cook for 30 minutes without lids, and stir occasionally.
2. In a bowl, serve with almond sliver, currants and remaining hemp seeds.

DELICIOUS QUINOA BREAKFAST CUP

Active time: 10 minutes
Cooking time: 40 minutes
Total time: 50 minutes
Yield: 6 servings

Protein: 7 grams per serving

Muffins are a breakfast you can easily eat anytime with their neat fillings. Another good thing about them is that you can enjoy them at your leisure.

INGREDIENTS:
- ½ 3 tablespoons cup plus quinoa
- 1/2 cup spinach
- Sliced mushroom ½ cup
- 1 cup milk
- 1/3 chickpea flour
- Nutritional yeast 1 tablespoon
- 2 tablespoons of raw
- 1/2 teaspoon salt

INSTRUCTIONS:
1. Sift the quinoa and rinse well. In a small pot, add quinoa and two tablespoons of water to one cup. Boil, cover and boil down. Cook for 10-15 minutes or until liquid is absorbed. Take it away from the heat and wait for 5 minutes with cover attached. Remove the lid and fluff.
2. Preheat oven to 375 ° F.
3. Put the muffin cup of paper in 6 cups of muffin tin.
4. Put the spinach and mushrooms in the food processor and process until finely chopped.
5. Add all ingredients to a large bowl and mix well.
6. Divide the mixture into muffin cups. Bake for 20-25 minutes.

CHAPTER FOUR

LUNCH RECIPES PEPITA AND ALMOND SQUARES

Active Time: 20 minutes
Cook Time: 15 minutes
Refrigerator Time: 30 minutes
Total Time: 1 hour 5 minutes
Yield: 16 squares

Protein: 12 grams per serving (2 squares)

Almonds and pepitas are two of the highest protein-packed seeds and nuts around. Combine them with even more powerhouse ingredients and you've got a very healthy little package.

INGREDIENTS

- 1 cup almonds, coarsely chopped
- 1 cup old-fashioned oats
- 2/3 cup pepitas
- 2/3 cup dried cranberries
- ½ cup unsweetened shredded coconut
- ¼ cup raw shelled hempseed
- 1/3 cup peanut butter
- 2/3 cup brown rice syrup
- ¼ cup maple syrup
- 2 teaspoons vanilla extract

INSTRUCTIONS

1. Line up a square baking tray with parchment paper and come up about 3 inches on opposite sides. This will act as a handle to remove the squares from the dish.

2. In a large mixing bowl, add the almonds, oats, pepitas, cranberries, coconut, and hempseed. Mix well. Stir in the peanut butter and try to get it evenly combined. You can use your fingers when most of it is worked in.

3. Add the brown rice syrup, maple syrup, and vanilla to a small saucepan. Bring to a boil and continue boiling until it reaches the hard ball stage, 260°F, on a candy thermometer. When this temperature is reached, quickly pour over the almond mixture and stir well. It will start to harden up quickly. Pour into the prepared dish and press down firmly into the dish and as evenly as possible. Refrigerate for at least 30 minutes.

4. Grab the "handles" of the parchment paper and lift out of the dish. Place on a cutting sheet and slice into sixteen squares.

LAYERED OAT AND CHOCOLATE BARS

Active Time: 20 minutes
Cook Time: 5 minutes

Refrigerator time: 1 hour Total Time: 1 hour 25 minutes
Yield: 16 squares

Protein: 7 grams per serving (1 square)

You wouldn't think that no-bake bars could look like this
and hold together like this, but they do. They're more like
a candy bar than anything else, except they're loaded with
protein.

INGREDIENTS
- 1 cup dairy-free butter
- ½ cup coconut sugar
- 1 teaspoon vanilla extract
- 3 cups quick-cooking oats
- ¼ cup raw shelled hempseed
- 2 tablespoons protein powder
- 1 cup dairy-free chocolate chips
- ½ cup peanut butter

INSTRUCTIONS
1. Position an 8 "square baking platter with baking
parchment paper and come up about 3 inches on opposite
sides. This will act as a handle to remove the squares from
the dish.
2. In a medium saucepan, melt the butter over medium-
high heat. Add the sugar and vanilla. Mix the in oats and
cook for 2 minutes. Add the hempseed and protein
powder and mix well. Pass half the mixture to the ready
one dish and press firmly and evenly into all edges and
corners.
3. Place the chocolate and peanut butter in a small
saucepan. Heat over low heat until chocolate is melted,
and all is well combined. Pour over the bottom layer in the
prepared dish and smooth evenly all over the top. Crumble

on top of what is left in the oat mixture as evenly as possible and lightly press into the chocolate.

4. Refrigerate for at least 1 hour. 5. Grab the "handles" of the parchment paper and lift out of the dish. Place on a cutting sheet and slice into sixteen squares.

CHOCOLATE CAKE MUNCH COOKIES

Active Time: 10 minutes
Refrigerator Time: 1 hour
Cook Time: 10 minutes
Total Time: 1 hour 20 minutes
Yield: 12 servings

Protein: 7 grams per serving (2 cookies)

Big, fat, and very chocolatey cookies are on the menu for today. Cake-like on the inside, they'll satisfy your cookie cravings any day.

INGREDIENTS

- ½ cup dairy-free butter, softened
- 1 cup coconut sugar
- 1 tablespoon chia seeds or ground chia seeds
- ¾ cup soy milk
- 1 teaspoon vanilla
- 2 cups whole wheat flour
- ¼ cup protein powder
- 1 teaspoon baking powder
- ½ teaspoon baking soda
- ½ teaspoon salt
- ½ cup cocoa powder
- 1 cup walnuts, chopped

INSTRUCTIONS

1. Stir in butter and sugar in a stand mixer tub. Mix on medium speed for 5 minutes.
2. Meanwhile, mix the chia seeds with 3 tablespoons water.
3. Add the chia mixture, milk, and vanilla to the butter and mix well at medium speed.
4. Add the flour, protein powder, baking powder, baking soda, salt, and cocoa to a medium bowl. Mix well.
5. Turn mixer on medium and slowly add the dry mixture. Add the walnuts and mix at low speed until combined. Place the mixture from 1 hour to overnight in the refrigerator.
6. About 15 minutes before you're ready to bake the cookies, preheat the oven to 400°F. Cut parchment paper on a baking sheet to match. put aside
7. Drop heaping tablespoons onto prepared cookie sheet, 2 inches apart. Roll into balls and then flatten by about half with the bottom of a measuring cup or some other strong material. They bake up thick. Bake for 8 minutes.
8. Cool on a wire rack.

CHOCOLATE SUNFLOWER PROTEIN COOKIES

Active Time: 15 minutes
Cook Time: 10 minutes
Total Time: 25 minutes
Yield: 12 servings

Protein: 7 grams per serving (2 cookies)

Sunflower seeds give these soft crunchy chocolate chip cookies a pleasant texture. Bake a few hundred for your belly and cookie jar.

INGREDIENTS
- 1 cup dairy-free butter
- ¾ cup plus 2 tablespoons coconut sugar

- 2 tablespoons ground chia seeds
- 2¼ cups whole wheat pastry flour
- ¼ cup protein powder
- 1 teaspoon baking soda
- ½ teaspoon baking powder
- ¼ teaspoon salt
- 1 teaspoon vanilla extract
- 1 cup dairy-free chocolate chips
- ¼ cup sunflower seed kernels

INSTRUCTIONS

1. Preheat to 375 ° F on burner. Cut parchment paper on a baking sheet to match. Set aside.
2. Add the butter and sugar to the stand mixer bowl and blend for 5 minutes at medium-low speed.
3. Meanwhile, mix and set aside ground chia seeds with 6 spoonfuls of water.
4. In a medium bowl, add the flour, protein powder, baking soda, baking powder, and salt.
5. Attach the combination of vanilla and chia to the butter blend. Mix well until blended. A little at a time, mix in the flour mixture. Mix the chocolate chips and the sunflower seeds at low speed.
6. Shape into round balls and set about 2 inches apart on the prepared baking sheet. Flat to approx. 1/2 inch high. Bake for 8 to 9 minutes.
7. Cool on a wire rack.

PEANUT BUTTER CHOCOLATE SEED BALLS

Active Time: 15 minutes
Refrigerator Time: 30 minutes
Cook Time: 25 minutes
Total Time: 1 hour 10 minutes
Yield: 16 servings

Protein: 7 grams per serving (3 balls)

Here are some perfect little bites that only have five ingredients. The delicious result gives you a nice firm ball. Simple and fast!

INGREDIENTS

- 16 ounces dairy-free chocolate chips
- ½ cup creamy peanut butter
- ½ cup raw shelled hempseed
- ½ cup unsweetened shredded coconut
- 1 cup sunflower seed kernels, pulsed fine in a mini food processor, divided

INSTRUCTIONS

1. Melt the chocolate in a double boiler. Stir in the peanut butter and blend well. Take off of the heat and mix in the hempseed, shredded coconut, and ½ cup sunflower seeds. Refrigerate until the dough is firm enough to use a small cookie scoop, about 30 minutes. 2. Remove the dough from the refrigerator and scoop out forty-eight balls. You can roll them into smoother balls with the palms of your hands. While they are still warm from rolling, roll them in the remaining pulsed sunflower seeds. 3. These will keep in the fridge for about 3 weeks and in the freezer for about 6 months.

PROTEIN POWER PISTACHIO BITES

Active Time: 15 minutes
Total Time: 15 minutes
Yield: 18 balls

Protein: 6 grams per serving (2 balls)

Who doesn't like pistachios? You can have these bites at a moment's notice, for yourself or friends. They're easy to pack along, too.

INGREDIENTS
- ½ cup old-fashioned oats
- ½ cup almond butter
- ¼ cup maple syrup
- 1/3 cup oat bran
- 1/3 cup flaxseed meal
- 1/3 cup pistachios, ground 1 tablespoon raw shelled hempseed

INSTRUCTIONS
1. Put all the ingredients in a big bowl and mix well.
2. Roll into eighteen balls.

TROPICAL LEMON PROTEIN BITES
Active Time: 20 minutes
Total Time: 20 minutes
Yield: 24 balls
Protein: 8 grams per serving (2 balls)

You have to have a lemon treat in your bag of tricks. Easy to make, these balls don't fall apart or make any kind of a mess.

INGREDIENTS
- 1¾ cups cashews
- ¼ cup coconut flour
- ¼ cup unsweetened shredded coconut
- 3 tablespoons raw shelled hempseed
- 3 tablespoons maple syrup
- 3 tablespoons fresh lemon juice

INSTRUCTIONS

1. Place the cashews in a food processor and process until very fine. Add the rest of the ingredients and process until well blended. Dump the mixture into a large bowl.
2. Roll the dough into solid small balls. Serve when ready.

NO-BAKE CEREAL DATE BARS

Active Time: 20 minutes
Cook Time: 15 minutes
Refrigerator Time: 30 minutes
Total Time: 1 hour 5 minutes
Yield: 16 bars
Protein: 9 grams per serving (2 bars)

Layers of crunchy goodness are filled with so many wonderful sweet flavors. Not too sweet, though—these bars have just the right contrast and balance.

INGREDIENTS

- 2 cups granola cereal
- 2 tablespoons flaxseed meal
- 2 tablespoons protein powder
- ½ cup peanuts, chopped
- ½ cup dates, chopped small
- ½ cup almond butter
- ½ cup brown rice syrup
- ¼ cup maple syrup

INSTRUCTIONS

1. Cover a square baking bowl with parchment paper and come up about 3 inches on opposite sides. This will act as a handle to remove the bars from the pan.
2. Combine the cereal, flaxseed meal, protein powder, peanuts, and dates in a large bowl.
3. In a small saucepan, add the almond butter and both syrups. Bring to a boil and cook to the hard ball stage, 260°F, on a candy

thermometer. Quickly stir into the cereal mixture and then spread into the prepared dish. It will cool quickly, so you can use your fingertips to press down into the dish as evenly as possible. Refrigerate for at least 30 minutes.

4. Grab the "handles" of the parchment paper and lift out of the dish. Put it on a cutting board and slice into 16 squares.

CHERRY CHOCOLATE HEMP BALLS

Active Time: 20 minutes
Total Time: 20 minutes
Yield: 24 balls
Protein: 10 grams per serving (2 balls)

Take a gander down this list of ingredients. Every nut, grain, fruit, and seed included here just makes one happy. They blend so well together and they freeze perfectly too.

INGREDIENTS

- 1 cup old-fashioned oats
- ½ cup unsweetened shredded coconut
- ½ cup dried cherries, chopped
- ½ cup pistachios, chopped
- 1/3 cup dairy-free chocolate chips
- 1/3 cup peanut butter
- ¼ cup maple syrup
- ¼ cup raw shelled hempseed

INSTRUCTIONS

1. Add all of the ingredients to a large bowl. Mix well with a sturdy wooden spoon. Roll into 24 balls.

2. Keep in the refrigerator for as long as 5 days or freeze for up to 6 months.

CHAPTER FIVE

DINNER RECIPES KALE THROW'S THREE-LAYER TACO

Active time: 25 minutes
Total time: 25 minutes
Yield: 3 servings

Protein: 30 grams per serving (2 tacos)

With these overflowing tacos, you'll want a taco night every night. The tofu is marinated with pinto beans and the spicy, sweet slaw acts as a topping.

INGREDIENTS:
Filling

- 1 tbsp taco seasoning
- 3 tablespoons
- 8 oz solid tofu, drainer, press, cut into ½ inch chunks
- 1 15 oz can focus, drain and rinse beans
- ¼ Cup fine onions
- Two diced roman tomatoes
- 1/2 teaspoon salt
- Pinch of ground black pepper
- 1 teaspoon chopped parsley

Kale Throw

- 1 cup coarsely chopped kale with stalks removed
- 1 tablespoon lemon juice
- 1 cup thin sliced purple cabbage
- 1 cup thinly sliced green cabbage
- ¼ cup carrot
- 2 tablespoons dairy free mayonnaise
- 1 tablespoon lime juice
- 1 tsp maple syrup
- 1 chopped pepper of finely chopped advo sauce

Assembly

- 6 taco shells

INSTRUCTIONS:

Filling

1. Mix taco seasoning and puddle in a small bowl. Set aside.

2. Add the tofu to the pool mix and toss. Marinate bean mixture and throw during work.

3. Put beans, onions, tomatoes, salt, hu pepper and parsley in a small bowl. Throw and melt. Kale Throw

4. Add kale to a medium bowl and add lemon juice. Massage the kale by hand to soften it. Add cabbage,

carrots, mayonnaise, lime juice, maple syrup and chili advo sauce. Mix well. Assembly

5. Assemble the tacos by layering the husks with a bean mixture, tofu and finally throw.

BREADED AND BAKED CAULIFLOWER TEMPETACOS

Active time: 15 minutes
Marinating time: 1 hour
Cook time: 30 minutes
Total time: 1 hour 45 minutes
Yield: 4 servings

Protein: 30 grams per serving (2 tacos)

The humble cauliflower has recently been in the spotlight for many good cooks, especially favored in this recipe. There are so many depths of flavors but this dish is still easy to pair.

INGREDIENTS:
- 8 oz original tempeh
- 3 tablespoons hot sauce (such as Frank)
- 1¼ cup and 2 tablespoons sugar-free dairy-free milk, split
- 1 small head cauliflower
- 1 cup whole wheat flour
- 2 tablespoons taco seasoning
- Panko bread crumb cup
- Nutritional yeast 2 tablespoons
- 1 tablespoon coconut oil
- Romaine lettuce 2 cups
- 8 taco shell

- 2 tomatoes, chopped
- Lime wedge (optional)
- Salsa (optional)

INSTRUCTIONS:
1. Preheat oven to 350 ° F.
2. Cut the tempeh into ¼-inch strips across the width and tear them into approximately ½-inch pieces.
3. Mix 1 tablespoon of hot sauce and 2 glasses of milk in a small bowl. Add tempeh and toss. Marinate for one hour.
4. Meanwhile, cut the small flowers into bite-sized pieces to prepare cauliflower.
5. Mix 2 tablespoons hot sauce and 1/4 cup milk in a large bowl. Add cauliflower and toss.
6. Add flour, taco seasoning, panko and nutritional yeast to a large bowl and mix well.
7. Remove the cauliflower from the wet mixture, add it to the flour mixture and coat all florets. Place on a baking sheet, bake for 20-30 minutes, spin after 15 minutes. When done, you can easily drill holes with a fork.
8. While baking the cauliflower, heat the oil in a small skillet over medium high heat and add tempeh. Cook for about 2 minutes, occasionally turn over and bake until the pieces turn golden. Move from heat to paper towel.
9. Put the lettuce on the bottom of the shell, put the tempeh, cauliflower and tomato with a spoon to assemble the taco. If needed, add lime wedges and salsa.

RICH MUSHROOM GRAVY AND POLENTA

Active time: 20 minutes
Cooking time: 45 minutes
Total time: 1 hour 5 minutes
Yield: 4 servings

Protein: 22 grams per serving

Polenta is rarely eaten despite being easy to make! Enjoy a meal with plenty of mushroom gravy.

INGREDIENTS:
Polenta

- ¼ cup coconut oil
- 1 tablespoon chopped shallot
- 3 pieces of garlic
- 1 teaspoon dried basil
- Dry white wine cup such as Chardonnay
- 3 cups vegetable soup
- chopped Roman tomato
- 1/2 teaspoon salt
- 1 cup cornmeal
- Mushroom gravy
- 2 tablespoons extra virgin olive oil
- 1 pound of button mushrooms, sliced
- 1 tablespoon chopped shallot
- 1 piece of garlic finely chopped
- 3 tablespoons flour
- 2 cups vegetable soup
- 1/2 teaspoon salt
- ¼ teaspoon ground black hu pepper
- 1 cup pressure cooker tender patties, crumbled

INSTRUCTIONS:
Polenta
1. Grease a 9-inch square pan.
2. Apply heat to the coconut oil in a big sauce pot over medium high heat. Add the shallots and cook for 3-5 minutes or until tender. Add the garlic and basil and cook. Stir the wine and bring to a boil. Reduce heat and cook for 5 minutes. Add soup, tomatoes and salt. Once it starts

boiling, lower the heat and add cornmeal. Cook and stir for 15-20 minutes or until the polenta has thickened and pulled off the side of the pan.

3. Pour into a ready pan and spread over in all four corners. Set aside for cooling to room temperature. This takes about 20-30 minutes. Mushroom gravy

4. Make mushroom gravy while the polenta is cooling. Drizzle olive oil in a frying pan. Add mushrooms and fry for 10-15 minutes. Add shallot and fry for 3-5 minutes. Add the garlic and flour and cook for another minute. Add vegetable soup, salt and pepper. Bring to a boil and then over medium heat, cook for about 5 minutes or until slightly thicker. Add the crushed putty, cook for another 5 minutes and heat.

5. Slice the polenta into squares and add 1-2 slices to a plate with mushroom gravy.

ARTICHOKE FLATBREAD WITH CRUSHED CITRUS

Active time: 20 minutes
Immersion time: 1 hour
Cooking time: 10 minutes
Total time: 1 hour 30 minutes
Yield: 2 servings

Protein: 39 grams per serving

You have to make this! Flatbread topped with these simple ingredients will bring a great deal of pleasure and healthy protein.

INGREDIENTS:
- Cashew cheese

- Soak the cup of raw cashew nuts for 1 hour to overnight and drain
- ½ cup of water
- Nutritional yeast 1 tablespoon
- 1 tablespoon tapioca starch or tapioca flour
- 1/2 teaspoon of garlic
- 1/2 teaspoon onion
- 1 tablespoon lemon juice

To assemble

- Two 8-inch flatbreads
- ¼ cup spinach, cut into strips
- Steamed Seitan Smoky Nugget in a cup
- 14 oz artichoke water
- 1 tomato, chopped
- ¼Canned sliced black olives in a cup
- Raw shelled cannabis for topping

INSTRUCTIONS:

Cashew cheese

1. Add all cheese ingredients to blender and mix until smooth. Turn this blended mixture into a saucepan. Cook over medium heat and stir until the sauce is slightly thicker. It takes 5-10 minutes. Let cool and take heat.

Assembly:

2. Spread a 1/2 cup layer of cashew cheese on each flatbread. Sprinkle half of the spinach on each flatbread. Separate citrus, artichoke, tomato and olives and sprinkle evenly on each flatbread.

3. Sprinkle on top with hemp seeds.

A COLLECTION OF THAI SEITAN AND VEGETABLES

Active time: 15 minutes
Cook time: 30 minutes
Total time: 45 minutes
Yield: 6 servings

Protein: 19 grams per serving

This is a multi-mix of all the best and most popular vegetables. Tasty citrus is added together with all the spices to make this jumbled pop flavorful.

INGREDIENTS:

- 2 carrots, sliced
- 1 small cauliflower cut into small flowers
- 1 small broccoli
- 1 tbsp extra virgin olive oil
- 1 diced white onion
- One red pepper, Julian
- 8 oz mushrooms, sliced
- 1 cup pressure cooker Thai nugget
- ¼ teaspoon time
- ¼ teaspoon basil
- ½ teaspoon salt
- ¼ teaspoon ground black pepper

INSTRUCTIONS:

1. Add water to a medium-sized pan with a steamer insert and bring to a boil. Add carrot and cauliflower and steam with boiling water for 5 minutes.

2. Add broccoli and cauliflower and steam for another 10 minutes. Pick all the vegetables and make sure they can be easily stabbed with a fork. Do not overheat. Al dente is best.

3. Apply heat the oil in a big saucepan. Add the onions and peppers and fry for 10 minutes. Position the mushrooms into the pan and boil for another 10 minutes. Add seitan

nuggets and all herbs and spices. Stir and heat for about 2 minutes. Add the cauliflower mixture, stir well and cook for another 5 minutes. Serve when hot.

SLOW COOKER POTATO TACOS

Active time: 15 minutes
Cooking time: 4 hours
Total time: 4 hours 15 minutes
Yield: 4 servings

Protein: 20 grams per serving (2 tacos)

Slow cookers can be a staple of the vegan household. The following is a list of easily found ingredients that can be dumped in to the slow cooker for an easy meal (excluding the tacos). There is no guessing what is included.

INGREDIENTS:
- Two 15 oz cans of beans, drained, rinsed
- 1 cup of fresh, frozen or canned corn
- 3 oz tipo pepper (approximately 2 peppers) in adobo sauce, chopped
- 6 oz tomato paste
- ¾Cup Thai sweet chili sauce
- 1 tablespoon sugar-free cocoa powder
- 1.5 tsp taco seasoning
- 8 white corn taco shells or tortillas or favorites
- Favorite toppings: spinach, lettuce, black olives, lime, avocado, peppers

INSTRUCTIONS:
1. Put everything except the taco shells and toppings into the slow cooker. Cook on low heat for 3-4 hours and on high heat for 1.5-2 hours.

2. Spread a considerable amount of filling on the taco shell. Add your favorite toppings.

BROCCOLI TOFU QUICHE

Active time: 30 minutes
Immersion time: 1 hour
Cooking time: 50 minutes
Total time: 2 hours 20 minutes
Yield: 6 servings

Protein: 21 grams of protein per serving

Elegance and protein are wrapped in this beautiful quiche. A special dinner full of vegetables and completely reheated. This quiche can be baked in a spring-foamed bread or pie dish.

INGREDIENTS:
Cashew cheese

- ¼ cup of raw cashew nuts, soaked for 1 hour
- ½ cup of water
- Nutritional yeast 1 tablespoon
- 2 tablespoons tapioca flour
- 1 tablespoon red miso
- 1/2 teaspoon cider vinegar
- 1/4 teaspoon salt
- ¼ teaspoon garlic powder

Quiche

- 1 tbsp extra virgin olive oil
- 1 cup spinach
- ½ red onion cup diced
- 1 cup of diced red peppers (about 1 pepper)
- 8 oz cremini mushrooms, sliced

- 1½ cup broccoli, the inner stem is cut into cubes, and the florets are cut into bites
- 3 pieces of garlic, finely chopped
- 1 cup of canned black beans, drain, rinse
- 16oz solid tofu, drained and pressed
- ¼ cup milk without dairy
- ¼ teaspoon turmeric
- 2 tsp oregano
- 1 tsp salt
- ¼ teaspoon ground black hu pepper
- One package vegan pie crust including two crusts

INSTRUCTIONS:

Cashew cheese

1. Add all cheese ingredients to the blender. Mix until smooth.

2. Pour into a small pot and cook on medium to high heat. It gets thicker and becomes slightly elastic within 5 minutes. If you think it is too thick to combine with the quiche ingredients, you can add one drop of water at a time. Set aside.

Quiche

3. Preheat oven to 350 ° F.

4. Heat the oil over medium heat in a large skillet. Add the spinach and cook until wilted. Remove from bread and set aside. Add the onions, peppers, mushrooms and broccoli to the pan and fry for about 10-15 minutes until the onions are translucent. Position the garlic and boil for two minutes and add black beans and stir. Pour into a large mixing bowl.

5. Divide the tofu into a blender and add milk, cashew cheese, turmeric, oregano, salt and pepper. Blend as smoothly as possible. Add the mixture to the stir-fried vegetables and mix well.

6. Pour into one pie crust. Cover with a second pie crust and crimp the ends. If using a spring foam pan, make a

rounded edge on the bottom skin and place the top skin on top of the material. Bake the quiche for 30 minutes.

PANDAN SEITAN CURRY

Active time: 20 minutes
Cooking time: 45 m minutes
Total Time: 1 hour 5 minutes
Yield: 6 servings

Protein: 26 grams of protein per serving

Add all of the peanut sauce, red curry paste and a small amount of hot sauce to make the key elements of this citrus and vegetable feast into a sweet and spicy medley.

INGREDIENTS:

- 1 cup red quinoa
- 1 sweet peeled potato that is cut into pieces
- 1 tbsp extra virgin olive oil
- 1 red pepper diced
- ¼ finely chopped shallots
- 2 garlic cloves
- ¼ cup creamy peanut butter
- 2 tablespoons red curry paste
- 1 teaspoon of Sriracha
- 2 tsp turmeric
- 1 teaspoon of raw g
- 1 teaspoon cumin
- 14 oz can coconut cream
- 1 tablespoon lime juice
- 1/2 teaspoon salt
- 2 cup pressure cooker Thai nuggets

INSTRUCTIONS:

1. Sift the quinoa and rinse well. Put the quinoa in a medium pot and cover with 2 cups of water. Bring to a boil and then reduce heat to cover. Cook for about 15-20 minutes or until all the water is absorbed and the quinoa is soft. Set aside and covered.

2. Add water to a medium-sized pan with a steamer and bring to a boil. Add the sweet potato to the insert and steam in boiling water for 10 minutes.

3. Apply heat to the oil in a big mixing skillet over average heat. Add peppers and fry for 10 minutes. Add shallot and garlic and cook for 2 minutes. Add peanut butter, red curry paste, sriracha, turmeric, ginger and cumin. Cook for 5 minutes, stirring occasionally. Add 1 cup of water, coconut cream, lime juice and salt and mix. Add sweet potatoes and sycamore nuggets. Stir to medium heat. Reduce boiling and cover the fire with low heat. Cook for 10-15 minutes.

4. Serve with quinoa.

MULTI-LAYER AVOCADO TOAST

Active time: 15 minutes
Cooking time: 5 minutes
Total time: 20 minutes
Yield: 2 servings

Protein: 16 grams per serving

Avocado toast is a popular option for brunch. Toasts topped with protein, fiber, and flavor make a simple breakfast to fuel your mornings.

INGREDIENTS:

- 1 tablespoon dairy-free butter
- 4 oz firm tofu, drained and pressed
- ¼ teaspoon black salt
- ¼ teaspoon onion powder
- Turmeric pinch

- 1 avocado
- Pinch of ground black pepper
- 1 teaspoon lime juice
- 2 slice sprouted grain bread

INSTRUCTIONS:

1. Add butter to a frying pan and heat over medium high heat. Crush the tofu in a frying pan. Sprinkle salt, onion powder and turmeric for about 4 minutes to make sure the tofu is broken into small pieces.

2. Using a medium bowl, crush the avocado with pepper and lime juice.

3. Toast the bread. Spread half of the prepared avocado on each part of the toast. Top with half of the prepared tofu on each piece of toast. Slice the toast diagonally in half.

SOUTHWEST SCRAMBLE BREAKFAST BURRITO

Active time: 10 minutes
Cooking time: 15 minutes
Total time: 25 minutes
Yield: 2 servings

Protein: 41 grams per serving

This recipe is a step beyond scrambled tofu. Add the vegetables and spices in 5 minutes and wrap it with the tortillas. The result is both filling and special.

INGREDIENTS:

- 1 tablespoon dairy-free butter
- ½ red pepper diced in a cup
- ½ red onion cup diced
- 8 oz firm tofu, drained and pressed

- ½ Cup steamed citrus potato rinks, crushed
- 1 tbsp taco seasoning
- 1/2 teaspoon salt
- 2 tablespoons flax seed meal
- 2 large tortillas with germinated grains

INSTRUCTIONS:

1. Apply heat to butter in a big mixing skillet over average high heat. Add peppers and onions and fry for 10 minutes. Crush the tofu with the prepared seitan. Stir for another 5 minutes, add taco seasoning and salt. Sprinkle the flaxseed meal and mix well.

2. Spoon half of the mixture into each tortilla and roll into a burrito. Cut in half and serve.

CHOCOLATE BANANA HEMP SMOOTHIE BOWL

Active time: 10 minutes
Total time: 10 minutes
Yield: 1 serving

Protein: 23 grams per serving

This is a good way to hide a little spinach in a chocolate banana smoothie bowl. Make it for breakfast to get a good start to the day.

INGREDIENTS:

Smoothie bowl

- 1 frozen banana, 4 slices for topping
- ½ cup almond milk or other dairy-free milk
- 1 tablespoon almond butter
- 1 tablespoon cocoa powder
- 1 tablespoon maple syrup

- 1 cup spinach

Toppings:

- 4 banana slices (from above)
- Strawberries and slices
- 2 tablespoons dairy-free chocolate chips
- 2 tablespoons of raw

INSTRUCTIONS:

1. Add the smoothie bowl ingredients in the blender and blend until smooth.
2. Pour into a bowl and decorate with toppings.

GRANOLA WITH SEEDS, NUTS AND FRUITS

Active time: 10 minutes
Cooking time: 40 minutes
Total time: 50 minutes
Yield: 8 servings

Protein: 16 grams per serving

This recipe can be stored in abundant quantities for about a month. Cereals stuffed with protein in the morning are a great way to start the day, especially if preparation is as easy as pouring into a bowl. With plant-based milk, you can add even more protein.

INGREDIENTS:

- 7 cups of traditional oats (use gluten free if needed)
- 1 cup shredded coconut
- 1 cup sunflower seed kernel
- 1 cup walnut
- 1 cup coconut sugar
- ¼ Cup chia seed
- 1 cup coconut oil

- 1 cup raisin

procedure:
1. Preheat oven to 300 ° F.
2. Mix all ingredients except raisins. Spread into a large baking pan.
3. Bake for 40 minutes. Remove from the oven and stir every 10 minutes. Return to the oven.
4. After 30 minutes, add the raisins and stir. Bake for another 10 minutes. Remove from oven and let cool.
5. Put in an airtight container. Keep for up to 4 weeks.

HIGH PROTEIN CHOCOLATE BLENDER MUFFIN

Active time: 15 minutes
Cooking time: 20 minutes
Total time: 35 minutes
Yield: 6 servings

Protein: 14 grams per serving (2 muffins)

These soft chocolate muffins are almost guilt-free! Blend, pour and bake for an easy way to consume chocolate protein.

INGREDIENTS:
- 1 15 oz black beans, drain, rinse
- ½ cup of apple sauce
- 2 tablespoons
- ¼ cup milk without dairy
- 1 tablespoon lemon juice
- ½ cup maple syrup
- 2 teaspoons of vanilla essence
- 1 tablespoon flax seed

- ½ cup of unsweetened cocoa powder
- 1 teaspoon baking powder
- 1/2 teaspoon baking soda
- ½ cup of traditional oats
- ½ choppedd dairy free chocolate chips
- ¼ cup raw cannabis with shell

INSTRUCTIONS:
1. Preheat oven to 350 ° F.
2. Line up the paper liner in a 12-cup muffin can.
3. Put all ingredients except chocolate chips and hemp seeds into the blender. Blend until the mixture is as smooth as possible. Add the chocolate chips and hemp seeds and mix for 5 seconds or until dispersed.
4. Pour into muffin cups and fill at least three quarters. Bake for 20 minutes. After cooling for 5 minutes, move the paper cup to a wire rack to cool completely.
5. Store in refrigerator for up to 3 days or freeze for up to 6 months.

LEMON STRAWBERRY PROTEIN MUFFIN

Active time: 15 minutes
Cooking time: 25 minutes
Total time: 40 minutes
Yield: 6 servings

Protein: 10 grams per serving (1 muffin)

This is a classic fat-free muffin recipe for satiety and satisfaction. Strawberry is added for a contrasting fruity touch that we all covet many times.

INGREDIENTS:

- 2 tablespoons crushed chia seed or chia seed, split
- 5 tablespoons butter without dairy
- ½ cup coconut sugar
- ½ cup + 2 tablespoons dairy free milk
- 1 tablespoon lemon juice
- 1.5 cups whole wheat flour
- 1.5 teaspoons of baking powder
- 1/2 teaspoon baking soda
- 1/4 teaspoon salt
- ¼ cup raw cannabis with shell
- ½ strawberry, chopped

INSTRUCTIONS:
1. Preheat oven to 375 ° F.
2. Grease the inside of a 6-cup muffin pan and set aside.
3. Mix 1 tablespoon ground chia seeds and 3 tablespoons water and save.
4. Using an electric mixer, mix the butter and sugar in a large bowl for about 3 minutes until lightly fluffy. Position the chia seed mixture and stir again while adding milk and lemon juice. Mix well.
5. Add flour, baking powder, baking soda, salt, cannabis, and the remaining tablespoon of chia seeds to a medium bowl. mixture. Put the flour mixture to the saturated mixture and tap until just bonded. It becomes a sticky batter. Fold the strawberries in. 6. Divide the batter into muffin cups. Fill at least three quarters, even if one cup is underfilled. Bake for 25 minutes, or until the toothpick inserted in the center is clean.

CRAZY QUINOA PROTEIN MUFFIN

Active time: 15 minutes
Cooking time: 35 minutes

Total time: 50 minutes
Yield: 6 servings

Protein: 7 grams per serving (1 muffin)

These cute muffins are crispy on the outside and cake-like on the inside. Sweeten with raisins and maple syrup to enjoy anytime.

INGREDIENTS:

- ½ Cup quinoa
- 2 tablespoons chia seeds
- ¼ cup almond flour
- 3 tablespoons of vanilla protein powder
- 1/2 teaspoon salt
- ½ Cup date, small increments
- 2 tablespoons coconut oil
- 3 tablespoons maple syrup
- 1 teaspoon of vanilla essence
- ¼ cup of unsweetened shredded coconut
- ½ cup raisins

INSTRUCTIONS:

1. Rinse the quinoa and put it in a small pot with a lid. Cover with a cup of water and boil over medium high heat. Cover and lower. Cook for 20 minutes and remove from heat. Remove the lid and let it cool.
2. Preheat oven to 450 ° F. Line up six muffin cups and paper liners.
3. Mix the ground chia seeds with ¼ cup and 2 tablespoons of water and save.
4. Add almond flour, protein powder and salt to a small bowl. Mix well. Add the date and mix on the coat. Set aside.
5. Put the coconut oil in a medium bowl. If not liquid, heat in a microwave for 10-20 seconds or until dissolved.

Remove from microwave and add maple syrup. Stir well. When cool, add the chia seed mixture, vanilla extract, coconut and almond flour mixture, cooked quinoa and raisins. Mix well.

6. Divide the batter between the six muffin cups and bake for 12-15 minutes until the nail p branch inserted in the center is clean.

FRESH VEGGIE SEITAN PITA POCKET

Active Time: 15 minutes
Cook Time: 5 minutes
Total Time: 20 minutes
Yield: 2 servings

Protein: 35 grams per serving

Fresh vegetables and tender seitan fill up these pita pockets for a memorable lunch.

INGREDIENTS
- 1 tablespoon extra-virgin olive oil
- 1 cup Steamed Seitan Smoky Nuggets, sliced thick
- ½ cup broccoli florets, chopped small
- ½ cup diced red bell pepper
- ½ cup diced cucumber
- 1 carrot, grated
- 4 ounces artichoke hearts in water, drained
- 2 pita pockets
- ¼ cup dairy-free mayonnaise
- 1 oz baby spinach

INSTRUCTIONS:
1. Steam the oil in a big saucepan over moderate to high steam. Add the seitan, broccoli, and bell pepper and cook

over medium heat for 3 minutes. Add the cucumber, carrot, and artichoke hearts. Stir and cook for 1 minute. Take off the heat.

2. Cut the pita pockets in half and spread half the mayonnaise into both halves of each pocket. Include baby spinach leaves and then spoon a quarter of the seitan mixture into each of the four pocket halves.

BROCCOLI SPINACH STUFFED BAGUETTE

Active Time: 45 minutes
Soaking Time: 1 hour
Cook Time: 25 minutes
Total Time: 2 hours 10 minutes
Yield: 2 servings

Protein: 31 grams per serving

A soft gooey cashew cheese with broccoli and spinach is added. Fill up a hollowed out baguette and it's a feast.

INGREDIENTS
Vegetables

- 2 cups of broccoli flower
- 1 tablespoon of extra virgin olive oil
- 2 cloves of garlic, finely diced
- 5 ounces of baby spinach, sliced, with long stems cut away and discarded
- Cashew Cheese ½ cup of raw cashew, soaked 1 hour and drained
- 1 cup of water
- ½ teaspoons of nutritional yeast
- 4 tablespoons of tapioca ½ teaspoon of salt
- ½ teaspoon of garlic powder

To prepare 1 baguette and 1 ounce of grapefruit

INSTRUCTIONS

1. Add water with a steamer applied to a medium saucepan and bring to a boil. Add the broccoli to the pipe, and steam 10 minutes over boiling water. Remove, and set aside from the steamer.
2. Steam up the oil over medium to high heat in a large skillet. Use a skillet that comes with a top. Add the garlic and boil for 1 minute. Stir in the spinach, toss, and simmer 1 minute. Cover for 2 minutes and let sit.
3. Remove the spinach and broccoli to a large bowl.
4. Apply all the ingredients of cashew cheese to a blender and combine until completely smooth.
5. Pour into a small saucepan and add medium - high pressure. Keep cooking and stirring until its thickening process is complete and becomes a gooey, salty sauce. It takes between 5 and 10 minutes.
6. Add the broccoli mixture to the pot. Shake it well.
7. Cut off the baguette top and use a spoon to scoop out some of the bread from the bottom. Make sure you leave a bread edge inside the shell to help hold the filling.
8. Spoon the broccoli-cheese mixture into the baguette core. Using sliced grape tomatoes to cover and scatter with hempseed. Half-cut. You may cut into slices as well and serve as an appetizer

TORTA DE SEITAN AND VEGGIES

Active Time: 45 minutes
Cook Time: 25 minutes
Total Time: 1 hour 10 minutes
Yield: 4 servings

Protein: 31 grams per serving

It can be difficult to not take samples straight form the skillet when this spicy mix is being prepared. Fill up those rolls and have a great lunch.

INGREDIENTS

- 1 tablespoon coconut oil
- ½ cup diced red onion
- 1 green bell pepper, diced
- 2 cloves garlic, minced
- ½ teaspoon dried oregano
- ½ teaspoon ground cumin
- 4 Steamed Seitan Chipotle Links
- 1 15 oz black beans, drain, rinse
- 2 sub rolls
- 1 cup salsa
- Romaine lettuce, sliced and chopped

INSTRUCTIONS

1. Heat up the oil over medium to high temperature in a large skillet and Stir in the onion and bell pepper and sauté for 10-15 minutes or until golden brown.

Stir in the garlic, oregano, cumin and roast for 1 minute. Tear the seiten into chunks and drop into the skillet. Add the black beans. Stir and cook over medium heat for 5 minutes or until seitan is heated through.

2. Halve each roll and chop out some of the bread center. Spread a layer of salsa on the bread and sprinkle on some chopped romaine lettuce. Fill up with black bean and seitan mixture.

SPROUTED GRAIN SPICY SEITAN SANDWICH

Active Time: 5 minutes
Cook Time: 10 minutes
Total Time: 15 minutes
Yield: 6 servings

Protein: 15 grams per serving

This super simple sandwich stars tender patties from an Instant Pot or pressure cooker. Make the seitan beforehand and keep in the fridge or freezer for a super-fast lunch.

INGREDIENTS
1 tablespoon coconut oil

- 6 Pressure Cooker Tender Patties
- 6 sprouted grain English muffins, sliced open
- Condiments of your choice, such as dairy-free chipotle mayo and horseradish mustard
- 1 avocado, sliced
- 6 slices red onion

INSTRUCTIONS
1. Steam the oil in a big skillet over an average-high heat and fry the patties until just golden on each side.
2. While the patties are in the skillet, toast the English muffins. Layer the toast with mayo, mustard, avocado, patty, and onion.

AMAZING LENTIL ENERGY BALLS

Active Time: 15 minutes
Refrigerator Time: 30 minutes
Cook Time: 25 minutes
Total Time: 1 hour 10 minutes
Yield: 9 servings

Protein: 12 grams per serving (4 balls)

What?! Lentil balls as a sweet protein snack? Yes, it's possible. In this recipe, they're sweetened just right—try them once and you'll be craving them forever. No kidding!

INGREDIENTS

- ½ cup lentils
- ½ cup dairy-free chocolate chips
- 2 cups quick-cooking oats
- ¼ cup sunflower seed kernels
- ¼ cup raw shelled hempseed
- ¼ cup unsweeted shredded coconut
- ½ cup almond butter
- ½ cup maple syrup

INSTRUCTIONS

1. Rinse lentils and drain them. In a medium-large saucepan, place 1 cup of water and the lentils. After high heat bring to a boil. Turn down to medium height when the water comes to boil and cook for 25 minutes or until the lentils are soft. We should consume all of the vapor. Set aside to freshen up.

2. In a large bowl incorporate the chocolate chips, peas, sunflower seeds, hempseeds, and coconut. Add in refrigerated lentils. Add the butter for almond and the maple syrup. Blend well. Shape into thirty-six balls and put them with a lid in a glass container.

3. Chill for about 30 minutes. Store for up to 5 days in the refrigerator or freeze for up to 6 months.

CHAPTER SIX

QUICK SNACKS

CHOCOLATE TRAIL MIX BARS

Active Time: 20 minutes
Refrigerator Time: 30 minutes
Total Time: 50 minutes
Yield: 8 bars

Protein: 16 grams per serving (1 bar)

These big and sturdy bars are great for the trail or even for just sitting in the backyard. Melted chocolate is included so they are nice and chocolatey too.

INGREDIENTS

- ¾ cup old-fashioned oats
- ½ cup bran flakes cereal
- ½ cup mixed nuts, chopped
- ¼ cup dried cherries
- ¼ cup dried cranberries
- ¼ cup raw shelled hempseed
- 3 tablespoons peanut butter
- ¼ cup maple syrup
- ½ cup dairy-free chocolate chips, melted

INSTRUCTIONS

1. Position an 8" square baking platter with baking parchment paper and come up about 3 inches on opposite sides. This will act as a handle for easy transferring of the bars.
2. Add the oats, cereal, nuts, cherries, cranberries, and hempseed to a large bowl and mix well.
3. Mix peanut butter with syrup together and move to the large bowl. Mix well. Fold in the melted chocolate .
4. Press firmly into the prepared dish and into all corners. Allow to cool in the refrigerator for 30 minutes. 5. Grab the "handles" of the parchment paper and lift out of the dish. Place on a cutting board and slice down the center. Turn and make three even cuts, which will give you eight long bars.

VANILLA ALMOND DATE BALLS

Active Time: 20 minutes
Total Time: 20 minutes
Yield: 20 balls

Protein: 8 grams per serving (2 balls)

Vanilla is such a great flavor, and it seems to make something a treat without going over the top. Almond flour and protein powder are added for an extra oomph of protein.

INGREDIENTS

- 1½ cups almond flour
- 16 dates, pitted
- 4 tablespoons sunflower seed kernels
- 4 tablespoons vanilla protein powder
- 2 tablespoons flaxseed meal
- 1 teaspoon vanilla extract
- Pinch of salt
- 2 tablespoons sunflower seed kernels, ground fine in a small food processor

INSTRUCTIONS

Excluding the ground sunflower seeds, place all ingredients in a food processor. Process on high until all is combined well and forms a ball. Move to a big bowl and form twenty balls. This dough works well by squeezing each repeatedly to form a ball. Roll in ground sunflower seeds.

ORANGE CRANBERRY POWER COOKIES

Active Time: 15 minutes
Cook Time: 10 minutes
Total Time: 25 minutes

Yield: 12 servings

Protein: 6 grams per serving (2 cookies)

This cookie has a refreshing flavor profile with hints of fruitiness and sweet cookie dough. Just one bite and it'll feel like they were made for special events only!

INGREDIENTS
- 1 cup dairy-free butter, softened
- 1 cup coconut sugar
- 1/3 cup orange juice
- 2 teaspoons organic vanilla extract
- 1½ cups whole wheat flour
- 2 tablespoons protein powder
- 1 teaspoon baking powder
- ¼ teaspoon baking soda
- 1 cup old-fashioned oats
- 1 cup dairy-free chocolate chips
- 1 cup walnuts, chopped
- 1 cup dried cranberries

INSTRUCTIONS
1. Preheat the oven to 375°F.
2. In a stand mixer dish, pound the butter and sugar together while adding the orange juice and vanilla extract. Mix well.
3. Mix dry ingredients in a medium bowl. Mix well with the wet mixture. Add the oats, chocolate chips, walnuts, and cranberries. Mix on low.
4. Drop heaping tablespoons about 2 inches apart on a baking tray. These are big cookies. They spread out to 3 to 4 inches in diameter. Bake for 10 to 11 minutes.
5. A few minutes after baking, transfer to a wire rack to cool completely.

RAW DATE CHOCOLATE BALLS

Active Time: 20 minutes
Refrigerator Time: 30 minutes
Total Time: 50 minutes
Yield: 24 balls

Protein: 6 grams per serving (2 balls)

These perfect little bites are made with the best variety of ingredients. They are sweet, crunchy, and chocolaty.

INGREDIENTS

- ¾ cup sunflower seed kernels, ground
- ½ cup dates, pitted, chopped well
- ½ cup walnuts, chopped
- ½ cup unsweetened cacao powder
- ½ cup maple syrup
- ½ cup creamy almond butter
- ½ cup old-fashioned oats (use gluten-free if desired)
- ¼ cup raw shelled hempseed
- 6 ounces unsweetened coconut, for coating

INSTRUCTIONS

1. Place the sunflower seeds, dates, walnuts, cacao powder, maple syrup, almond butter, oats, and hempseed in a large bowl. Mix well.

2. Cut the dough into pieces and wrap into twenty-four balls. Roll each ball in shredded coconut. It will harden in 30 mins in the refrigerator.

PACKED PEANUT OATMEAL COOKIES

Active Time: 15 minutes
Cook Time: 11 minutes

Total Time: 26 minutes
Yield: 12 servings

Protein: 8 grams per serving (2 cookies)

Peanuts, oats, and dairy-free cream cheese are just the beginning of making a classic cookie that's packed with protein. What's more, they hardly take any time to make!

INGREDIENTS
- 1 tablespoon chia seeds or ground chia seeds
- 1 cup whole wheat flour
- 1 teaspoon baking powder
- 1½ cups old-fashioned oats
- 2 tablespoons vanilla protein powder
- ½ cup dairy-free butter
- 1 cup coconut sugar
- ½ cup dairy-free cream cheese, softened
- 1 teaspoon vanilla extract
- 1 banana
- 1 cup peanuts, chopped

INSTRUCTIONS
1. Preheat the oven to 400°F
2. Mix the chia seeds with 3 tablespoons water and set aside.
3. Add the flour, baking powder, oats, and protein powder to a large bowl. Set aside.
4. In the mixer, add the butter and sugar. Cream on medium-low speed for 5 minutes. Mix in the cream cheese well. Turn off the beater and add the prepared chia seed mixture, vanilla, and banana. Mix well on medium speed. Add the flour mix and peanuts and keep mixing until just combined.

5. Spoon dollops on the baking tray, 2 inches apart. You can use a glass-bottom to flatten the cookie to ½-inch thick. Bake for 11 minutes.
6. Cool on a wire rack.

CHOCOLATE CHIP BANANA BREAD PROTEIN COOKIES

Active Time: 15 minutes
Cook Time: 15 minutes
Total Time: 30 minutes
Yield: 12 servings

Protein: 6 grams per serving (2 cookies)

These protein-rich cookies are high in fiber which keeps you feeling full and satisfied. They taste delicious too!

INGREDIENTS

- 2 tablespoons of chia seed or ground chia seed
- 1 cup whole wheat flour
- ½ cup almond flour
- ½ cup flaxseed meal
- 2 tablespoons protein powder
- ½ teaspoon baking soda
- ½ teaspoon salt
- ¾ cup dairy-free butter
- 2/3 cup coconut sugar
- 1/3 cup organic light brown sugar, packed
- 1 teaspoon vanilla extract
- ½ cup banana, mashed (1 medium banana)
- 1 cup dairy-free chocolate chips

INSTRUCTIONS

1. Preheat the oven to 350°F. Cut parchment paper on a baking sheet to match. Put aside.
2. Mix the chia seeds with 6 tablespoons of water and set aside.
3. To the large bowl, add both flours, and other dry ingredients. Set aside.
4. Add butter to the mixer bowl, including sugars. Mix on medium speed for 5 minutes. Switch off beater then add the mixture of chia seeds, cinnamon and banana to cook. Mix well to low velocity. Add the dry ingredients and start to mix until just combined. Clear the chocolate chips from and fold in mixing bowl and fold.
5. Place heaping tablespoons on a cookie sheet 2 inches apart and flatten with the bottom of a glass to about ½ inch thick. Bake for 12 minutes.
6. Cool on a wire rack.

CRUNCHY NUTS AND SEEDS PROTEIN BARS

Active Time: 15 minutes
Refrigerator Time: 30 minutes
Total Time: 45 minutes
Yield: 16 bars

Protein: 9 grams per serving (1 bar)

A little miracle happens after these bars cool. They turn into a caramel-like bar that gives satisfaction to no end. Chocolaty and chewy!

INGREDIENTS
- 2 cups chickpea flour
- 1 cup plus 2 tablespoons almond flour
- 2 tablespoons flaxseed meal
- 1 cup dairy-free milk

- 1 cup cashew butter
- ½ cup maple syrup
- ½ cup slivered almonds
- ½ cup dried cranberries
- ¼ cup sunflower seed kernels
- ½ cup dairy-free chocolate chips, melted

INSTRUCTIONS

1. Cover the square baking bowl with parchment paper and come up about 3 inches on opposite sides. This will act as a handle to remove the bars from the dish.

2. Combine the dry mix in a large bowl and mix well. With a heavy wooden spoon, mix in the milk, cashew butter, maple syrup, almonds, cranberries, and sunflower seeds. Lastly, mix in the liquid chocolate. Add the batter to the prepared dish and press firmly into all corners and as evenly as possible. Refrigerate for at least 30 minutes.

3. Grab the "handles" of the parchment paper and lift out of the dish. Place on a cutting sheet and slice into sixteen bars.

OVER-THE-TOP BARS TO GO

Active Time: 20 minutes
Refrigerator Time: 30 minutes
Cook Time: 15 minutes
Total Time: 1 hour 5 minutes
Yield: 16 squares

Protein: 13 grams per serving (2 squares)

Not only are these bars gorgeous, they travel really well too. The ingredients are fun because they contain just about every nut and seed that you can think of.

INGREDIENTS

- 1½ cups rolled oats
- ½ cup pecans
- ½ cup pistachios
- ½ cup cashews
- ½ cup dried cranberries
- ¼ cup dates, pitted and chopped
- ¼ cup sunflower seed kernels
- ¼ cup pepitas
- 2 tablespoons raw shelled hempseed
- ½ cup peanut butter
- ½ cup brown rice syrup
- 3 tablespoons maple syrup

INSTRUCTIONS

1. Cover square baking bowl with parchment paper and come up about 3 inches on opposite sides. This will act as a handle to remove the bars from the dish.

2. Excluding peanut butter and both syrups, mix everything together. Gradually mix peanut butter until incorporated, then use your hands to mix and pinch so that the peanut butter is well incorporated into the dry ingredients.

3. Add the brown rice syrup and maple syrup to a small saucepan. Bring to a boil and cook to hard ball stage, 260°F, on a candy thermometer. Pour the syrups in the mixture and stir well. Then quickly press the mix over the parchment paper. It will cool quickly, so you can use your fingertips to press down into the dish or use the bottom of a measuring cup to press down firmly. Refrigerate for at least 30 minutes.

4. Grab the "handles" of the parchment paper and lift out of the dish. Put on a cutting board and slice into 16 squares.

NO-BAKE CHOCOLATE PEANUT BUTTER COOKIES

Active Time: 5 minutes
Resting Time: 1 hour
Cook Time: 5 minutes
Total Time: 1 hour 10 minutes
Yield: 24 cookies

Protein: 7 grams per serving (2 cookies)

Although these are no-bake cookies, they have the texture of baked cookies. They have no refined sugar, take 10 minutes to make, and are a favorite. They deserve a five-star rating in our books!

INGREDIENTS

- ½ cup unsweetened dairy-free milk
- 3 tablespoons dairy-free butter
- 1/3 cup coconut sugar
- 1 tablespoon sugarfree cocoa powder
- 1/3 up dairy-free semi-sweet chocolate chips
- 1 teaspoon vanilla extract
- 1/3 cup creamy peanut butter
- Pinch of salt
- 2½ cups rolled oats or quick-cooking oats
- ¼ cup raw shelled hempseed

INSTRUCTIONS
1. Stack wax paper on a baking sheet.
2. Place the milk, butter, sugar, cocoa powder, and chocolate chips in a large saucepan. Put melt and boil slightly for 2 minutes. Stir occasionally so that the chocolate chips don't stick burn before they melt. Remove

from the heat. Mix in the vanilla, peanut butter, and salt until the peanut butter melts. Stir in the oats and hempseed.

3. Drop flour dollops onto the prepared baking sheet with one spoon. You will take them in a minute or less and transform them into cookies. Let the cookies set for around an hour. Placing them in the refrigerator can accelerate the cooling and hardening process.

APRICOT PISTACHIO ENERGY SQUARES

Active Time: 15 minutes
Cook Time: 10 minutes
Refrigerator Time: 30 minutes
Total Time: 55 minutes
Yield: 16 squares

Protein: 8 grams per serving (2 squares)

Every good flavor you can think of is in these perfect little squares. Besides heavenly apricot and dates, you have the option of drizzling chocolate over the top.

INGREDIENTS
- 1 ½ cups dates, pitted, chopped
- 1 cup dried apricots, chopped
- 1 cup cashews, chopped
- ½ cup old-fashioned oats
- ½ cup pistachios
- 3 tablespoons cashew butter
- 2 tablespoons ground ginger
- ½ cup brown rice syrup
- 2 tablespoons maple syrup
- 1 teaspoon vanilla extract

- ¼ cup dairy-free chocolate chips (optional)

INSTRUCTIONS

1. Position an 8" square baking platter with baking parchment that come up to about 3 inches on opposite sides. This will act as a handle to remove the squares from the dish.

2. Add the dates, apricots, cashews, oats, and pistachios to a large bowl. Mix in the cashew butter and ground ginger and combine as well as you can. You can use your fingers to help blend it all together.

3. In a small saucepan, add the brown rice syrup, maple syrup, and vanilla. Bring to a boil and continue boiling until it reaches the hard ball stage, 260°F, on a candy thermometer. Quickly add to the date mixture and mix well. Pour into the prepared dish and press firmly and evenly into all edges and corners. Chill in the cooler for at least 30 minutes.

4. Grab the "handles" of the parchment paper and lift out of the dish. Place on a cutting sheet and slice into sixteen squares. 5. If desired, melt the chocolate chips over the stove or in the microwave. Drizzle in a zig-zag motion over the bars.

HIGH-PROTEIN PEANUT BUTTER COOKIE DOUGH

Active Time: 15 minutes
Total Time: 15 minutes
Yield: 45 balls

Protein: 6¾ grams per serving (2 balls)

Here's a simple and delicious recipe. With minimal ingredients and about 15 minutes, you can have a delicious dessert.

INGREDIENTS
* 1 cup peanut butter (crunchy)
* 1 cup grade A maple syrup
* ½ teaspoon salt
* 1 cup chickpea flour
* ¾ cup almond meal flour
* ½ cup peanuts, chopped
* ½ cup cashews, chopped
* ½ cup old-fashioned oats
* Finely ground peanuts, for coating (optional)

INSTRUCTIONS
1. Mix the peanut butter and the syrup in a large bowl. Mix all other ingredients together well. Roll into bite-sized balls and they are ready to serve.
2. If you want a more elegant look, roll the balls into finely ground peanuts. Prolong shelf life by storing in the refrigerator between snacking.